Over 250 Ways To Cook And Serve Fish And Other Productions Of The Sea

A Choice Collection Of Recipes, Representing The Latest And Most Approved Methods Of Cooking

INTRODUCTION.

"There are many fishes in the Sea," in fact so many that it is possible to have a different kind served every day of the year, and still not exhaust the variety, but it is necessary to the attainment of this result to have the resources of a great city fish market at one's command. Thanks to the skill of the trained cook there are an infinite number of ways in which the commoner sort of fish that are to be had everywhere, can be transformed into a great variety of dainty, yet simple and inexpensive dishes. And here is the value of this publication.

Cook books there are of all sorts and shapes, but strange to say the subject of Fish Cookery has been sadly neglected in all of them, and to supply this deficiency, the following collection of receipts has been carefully gathered and properly arranged for the convenience of the housewife, no time or expense having been spared to make the volume a thoroughly reliable and practical guide upon the important subject which it treats.

The experience of distinguished chefs and epicures of many lands have been fully drawn upon, while noted travellers, anglers, and sportsmen, who have been pleased with the cookery of some famous guide or cook, have revealed his secrets for the benefit of our readers. The famous housekeepers have assisted, too, and have contributed generously from the wealth of their experience. In addition to the receipts there will be found within the covers of the book much other information of value to the reader, about the best fish foods, where obtained and how to be made of the best service. It is in every way a complete guide to the culinary art as applied to the fish family.

CAREINTHECOOKROOM.
ImportanceofSelectingtheBestintheLineofFoodSupplies.

Housekeepers throughout the land are every day becoming better informed regarding the relative quality of articles of food offered in the markets, and the tradesman who does not cater to this growing knowledge will soon lose the patronage of his best customers. People of intelligence now demand the best in food products, and the essential features of superiority insisted upon are palatableness, purity and wholesomeness. These qualities must unite in order that the stamp of approval may be bestowed, and a product lacking any one of these cardinal requirements cannot hope for lasting success. Upon the other hand, when any article of food supply has demonstrated that it not only pleases the taste, but is also nutritious and in every way conducive to health, the popularity of such product is assured.

An illustration of the preceding statement is happily furnished in the pronounced popularity of "Gold Wedge" Brand of Fibered Codfish, a product absolutely without odor, and requiring no boiling or soaking, which must be conceded a place of pre-eminence among the food products of unquestioned value now being offered. That this article possesses all the necessary qualifications for its acceptance by the most keenly critical and discriminating housekeeper has been so frequently and so thoroughly demonstrated that it is scarcely worth while to more than allude to such fact. That it has attained to the highest place in the confidence of consumers is ample proof of its superiority. The cardinal virtues of Palatableness, Purity and Wholesomeness have rendered "Gold Wedge" Brand of Fibered Codfish a favored article of food in refined and intelligent homes, and caused it to be regarded as a necessary part of the menu.

Wherever unquestioned worth in any food article is amply proved it is the duty of the physician to bestow his commendation, and hygienic publications should be foremost in extending their meed of praise, for to these two sources the general public must ever look for unbiased and competent advice upon all matters pertaining to the health and well-being of the people; it is, therefore, with more than ordinary pleasure that we bear testimony to the appetizing and wholesome qualities of "Gold Wedge" Brand of Fibered Codfish, which is in all respects worthy of highest praise.

The manufacturers of this superior food product, Shute & Merchant, Gloucester, Mass., are of such standing commercially that their brand is indicative of merit; and we feel no hesitancy in bestowing heartiest approval upon their wares. To those of our readers who have written us concerning this product, and to others who may not be fully conversant with the high qualities of the same, we would say that "Gold Wedge" Brand of Fibered Codfish is all that could be desired, and that it should find a place upon every table where the laws of health, as well as the gratification of the appetite, receive the proper consideration. Any first-class dealer will supply this article if insisted upon, and those catering to refined patronage will see the necessity of keeping it in stock.

J. W. ARNOLD, M. D.

GENERALINSTRUCTIONS.

To economize space and avoid much unnecessary repetition, we herewith append such directions for the treatment of fish preparatory to cooking as admit of general application.

No. 1. When a Fish is Fresh.—When the gills of a fish are of a bright color, and the eyes appear full and clear, it is quite fresh; if the flesh seems hard and firm and rises quickly from pressure with the finger, its freshness is still farther assured. Although a fish that will not stand these tests may not be spoilt, its goodness has deteriorated in proportion as it fails to meet such requirements, and it is so much less desirable for the table. The sense of smell cannot be relied upon to decide the question of freshness.

No. 2. To Dress or Clean a Fish.—Some fish require scaling and some need to be skinned before cooking. The sooner a fish is scaled after taking from the water, the easier it can be done. Some fish of the scaly variety, however, should never be scaled as the scales of such are esteemed a delicacy. Such exceptions will be noted in the recipes for cooking these fish. When the scales of a fish have become dry and hard or the fish is a difficult one to scale from any cause, it should be soaked for a while in cold salted water. If you have not time to do this, hold the fish up by the tail and pour boiling water over it, but do not let it lie in hot water for an instant. Having scaled the fish, the next question is how is it to be cooked? for this has much to do with the dressing process.

No. 3. To prepare for Baking or Boiling.—If the fish is a large one and to be cooked whole, it should be opened from the vent up as far as the ventral fins,—taking care not to mutilate the roes or livers if they are wanted for cooking. With a sharp knife separate the intestines from the body, also the gills from the head, and pull out all together through the natural gill opening. The reason for opening the fish as little as possible, is to keep it in best possible shape for stuffing, but if no stuffing is to be used the opening may be made larger to suit the convenience of dressing. When the gills and intestines have been removed, the fish should be washed freely in cold salted water, and all clotted blood thoroughly removed. Only under conditions hereinafter specified should fish be washed after the fins have been cut out or the solid flesh of the fish has been cut into. No washing of the flesh can make it any cleaner than it is in its natural condition, and if the fish is washed after the flesh has been cut you are simply bringing the slime and blood in contact with it, and the more you wash it the more you are rubbing it in, and the fish may become so impregnated as to be extremely strong when cooked. This is a point that should not be disregarded if you would have sweet-flavored fish. After washing thoroughly, wipe perfectly dry, then either cut out or trim off the fins, as occasion requires or tastes suggest. A pair of scissors will be found very convenient for trimming off the fins.

No. 4. To prepare Fish for Broiling.—Dress, wash and wipe dry before splitting. Always split a fish on the under side, and unless the fish is very small indeed remove the back bone entire, then the thickest part of the fish will come over the center and hottest part of the fire, and both sides will be cooked alike, whereas if the back bone is left in one side, that side will take longer to cook, and will be less desirable after it is cooked, for when the back bone is removed from the cooked fish a good part of the brown part is taken off with it, and it loses its flavor as a broiled fish. Properly broiled, all parts should be equally browned, both an account of flavor and appearance. Very small fish are sometimes broiled without splitting; these should be dressed the same as for frying.

No. 5. To prepare Fish for Frying.—Fish may be fried whole in steaks or fillets. Those to be fried whole must be dressed, then washed and wiped perfectly dry. Steaks are slices of fish cut crosswise; fillets are made from steaks or from pieces of fish cut off lengthwise, and may be any size or shape to suit individual tastes. The best way to make fillets is to dress and split the fish, remove the back bone and then cut the fish into halves, quarters or eights, according to size.

No. 6. Fish to Skin.—Fish that require to be skinned before cooking, should be first dressed and washed clean, then remove the skin, head, tail and fins, rinse quickly in clear cold water and wipe thoroughly dry.

☞ **Notice.**—No repetition of the foregoing directions for dressing and cleaning fish will occur in connection with any recipes to which they are applicable. When other treatment is requisite special directions will accompany the recipe.

No. 7. Fish Cookery in General.—Under this head will be found such instructions for the cooking of fish as are applicable to any or all kinds. Special recipes for special varieties are given elsewhere (see index) but many of these are equally suited to other fish of similar qualities.

No. 8. Fish to Fry.—Fish may be fried in olive oil, pork fat, lard, cottolene, or clarified drippings; the latter being probably the most economical; the first chiefly used in French or high-class cookery, but we favor pork fat ourselves. Whatever fat is used it should be deep enough to cover the fish and hot enough to brown a piece of bread handsomely in thirty seconds or less. The pork fat is made by trying out thin slices of fat salt pork, being careful not to let it burn. The pork gives the fish a flavor not to be obtained by the use of salt in connection with other oils or fats. When the pork fat is used salt should be used sparingly if at all. Fried fish should be seasoned while cooking. The slices of pork may be used as a garnish and served with the fish. After wiping dry, fish should be rolled in Indian meal, flour, cornstarch, or crumbs before frying. If the fish has been on ice or is very cold, do not put it into the fat fast enough to cool it perceptibly. Watch carefully while cooking, don't break or mutilate in turning or dishing, cook a nice brown, drain on a sieve, colander or paper, and serve hot on a napkin. Unless fish are very small they should be notched each side before rolling in meal or other absorbents previous to frying.

No. 9. To Saute, is to fry in just fat enough to cover bottom of frying pan.

No. 10. To Broil.—The process of broiling is probably the most simple as well as the most desirable method of cooking many kinds of fish, the natural flavor and juices being better preserved than by any other, and the flavor may be further enhanced by the judicious use of seasoning, herbs, etc., preparatory to broiling (see recipes for broiling.) The double iron broiler is unquestionably the best utensil for broiling fish, yet they may be broiled on a griddle or in a spider. Heat hot and butter well before laying in the fish, cook the flesh side first, when that is perfectly browned turn and finish cooking. Serve on a hot platter, spread with butter or cream or both and season to taste. A fish may also be broiled in a good hot oven in the dripping pan, and if it be a very fat one will cook nicely. The pan should be well buttered and the fish placed skin side down and cooked without turning. Basting once or twice with butter or cream while cooking is advisable.

No. 11. To Boil.—Boiling is considered by many the most insipid and undesirable way of cooking fish, yet there are certain varieties that are best cooked this way if accompanied by a rich sauce. The fish boiler is almost indispensable to success in boiling or steaming a whole fish, but everybody hasn't one, and to such we would say utilize the wash boiler. Put a bowl or something in each end that will support a platter, either side up; on the platter lay the fish and add water enough to reach the platter without coming in contact with the fish, thus enabling you to steam the fish, which is preferable to boiling. Fish boiled in a common kettle should first be wrapped closely in cheese cloth or fine muslin to preserve its shape. The head is the best part of a boiled fish, and the nearer the head the better the remaining portion. Boiled fish should be served on a napkin and the sauce in a tureen. A fish of six pounds should boil or steam in thirty or thirty-five minutes. The water should always be salted. A boiled fish may be stuffed, but usually they are not. Recipes for sauces suitable for boiled fish will be found under the head of sauces, (Nos. 13 to 56.)

No. 12. To Bake.—Different varieties of fish, different sizes, and different portions of fish require such varied treatment in baking we can offer but few general rules for this branch of cookery. Our recipes, however, will supply all needed information. A dripping pan with a false bottom, either wire or perforated, with a handle at each end by which to lift it, is particularly desirable in baking fish. Wanting these, strips of cloth well buttered and placed across the bottom of the pan will be found extremely convenient for lifting out the fish. A baked fish presents a more attractive appearance when served in an upright position on the platter, and also cooks much nicer in this condition. To keep it so while cooking, first press it down enough to flatten the under side, then if necessary brace it up with skewers or with potatoes placed against it until it is well under way for cooking, when it will keep its position until cooked and dished. Sometimes it is advisable to bend the fish half-moon shape and cook it that way, or if the fish is long and slender the tail may be tied to the mouth, either of which methods will keep the fish in upright position. Dressing and force-meats are considered elsewhere, and indexed under their appropriate headings.

☞ The secret of success in all kinds of fish cookery is to so cook and serve it that it shall be attractive in appearance and satisfying in flavor; that is, the flavor when especially agreeable or desirable must be retained or enhanced. When the flavor of a fish is insipid or unpleasant it must be cooked with a view to imparting an unnatural but at the same time pleasant flavor instead. This is the secret of success in fish cookery, and these points have been especially considered in the selection of the accompanying recipes.

No. 13. Sauces.—Sauces are extensively used in all kinds of fish cookery. For convenience in reference we have given them first place among our recipes. Although consommes or stocks are not absolutely indispensable in connection with fish cookery, they are nevertheless extremely useful in the making of nice sauces, and recipes for making them in great variety may be found in almost every cook book, still we have thought best to give directions for making two of those most frequently used in preparing the following sauces. When stocks are not at hand, liquor in which fish have been cooked will answer every purpose, and even milk or water, or both may be substituted.

No. 14. Consomme or White Stock.—A French method of making a white stock, is to put in a stock pot, or kettle, a roast fowl (chicken,) or the remains of a chicken or turkey, a knuckle of veal, say four pounds, one pound of beef and three quarts of water, when scum begins to rise skim carefully, until it ceases to appear, then add a carrot, a turnip, an onion, a leek, two cloves, two stalks of celery, and a little salt, simmer very gently four hours. Remove every particle of grease and strain through a flannel cloth, kept for the purpose.

No. 15. Fish Stock.—Two pounds of veal, four pounds of fish, or more veal, and less fish, if you do not have as much fish, two onions, rind of half a lemon, bunch sweet herbs, two carrots, two quarts water. Cut up fish and meat and put with other ingredients into the water, simmer two hours, skim liquor carefully and strain. When a richer stock is wanted, fry the vegetables and fish before adding the water.

No. 16. Drawn Butter.—No. 1. This is the simplest and most generally used of any fish sauce, and serves as the foundation for a large proportion of such sauces. It can be made very economically also, its cost depending upon the amount of butter used. Simple as it is many people fail in making it. To make it nice and smooth with one pint hot water, half a cup of butter, two teaspoons flour, half a teaspoon salt and half a saltspoon of pepper, put one-half the butter in a saucepan and melt without letting it brown, add the dry flour, mixing well, then stir in the hot water, a little at a time, stir rapidly as it thickens; when perfectly smooth add the remaining butter bit by bit and stir until all absorbed, then add the seasoning; if carefully made it will be free from lumps, if it is not smooth strain before serving.

No. 17. Drawn Butter Sauce.—No. 2. Pour boiling hot drawn butter sauce (No. 16) into the well beaten yolks of two eggs, mix thoroughly, season to taste, and serve quickly.

No. 18. Cream Sauce.—This sauce is made by substituting cream or milk for water in the drawn butter sauce (No. 16.)

No. 19. White or White Stock (No. 14) substituted for the water in drawn butter sauce (No. 16) makes this sauce.

No. 20. Acid Sauce.—Lemon juice or vinegar added to the drawn butter sauce (No. 16.)

No. 21. Anchovy Sauce.—Bone four anchovies and bruise in mortar to a smooth paste and stir them in a drawn butter sauce (No. 16,) simmer five minutes, or stir in two teaspoons of essence of anchovy. A little cayenne added is an improvement.

No. 22. Egg Sauce. To make this sauce add two or three hard boiled eggs, chopped or sliced, to the drawn butter sauce (No. 17.)

No. 23. Parsley Sauce.—Add two teaspoons of chopped parsley to the drawn butter sauce (Nos. 16 or 17.)

No. 24. Caper Sauce.—Add capers to suit to a plain drawn butter sauce (No. 16,) or to a White sauce (No. 19.)

No. 25. Hollandaise Sauce.—One cup of butter, yolks of two eggs, juice of half a lemon, one saltspoon of salt, pinch of cayenne, half a cup of boiling water. Rub butter to a cream, add yolks one at a time, and beat well, adding lemon juice, salt and pepper. A few minutes before serving add the boiling water, place the bowl in a saucepan of boiling water, and stir rapidly until it thickens like a boiled custard.

No. 26. Wine Sauce.—Mix and knead well together in a bowl two ounces of butter, one tablespoon of chopped parsley, juice of one-half a lemon, salt and pepper, speck of mace, and one wine glass of Madeira or sherry wine. Beat the butter to a cream and gradually beat in the seasoning. A tablespoon of vinegar may be substituted for the wine if preferred. This sauce is particularly nice for broiled fish. It should be poured over the fish.

No. 27. Cardinal Sauce.—Cardinal sauce is, as a rule, made from lobsters and colored with coral; so, if possible, purchase lobsters containing coral. Boil the lobster; open and remove the coral and press it through a sieve. Put two tablespoonfuls of butter into a pan; let it melt. Add a tablespoonful of flour mixed, without browning; add one-half pint stock, one-half teaspoonful of onion juice, and a bay leaf. Stir constantly until it boils. Take out the bay leaf; add a palatable seasoning of salt and pepper, the coral and a little of the red part of the lobster chopped fine and serve.

No. 28. Sauce Soubise.—Peel and chop three onions; simmer them with one ounce of butter for three quarters of an hour, but do not let them color very much. Add one tablespoon of flour, salt, pepper and a pinch of mace, and mix all together; moisten with half a pint of the fish liquor, and the same quantity of hot cream or milk. Serve in tureen.

No. 29. Shrimp Sauce.—Take half a pint of drawn butter or white sauce (No. 19) and when boiling add a little lobster coral, if you have it, if not, add half a teaspoon of anchovy essence. Remove the shells from four dozen shrimp, put them into the sauce, heat and serve. Canned shrimp may be substituted for the fresh.

No. 30. Lobster Sauce.—Take the meat from a boiled lobster weighing about one pound, cut it into dice-shaped pieces. Add two ounces of butter to the coral, rub it together with the blade of a knife, and press it through a sieve. Make a butter sauce with cream, put in the coral, season with salt, pepper and a little mace, and heat it hot without allowing to boil; add the lobster meat, let it get hot again without boiling, and serve in sauce tureen. If allowed to boil it will spoil its color, which is one desirable feature of this sauce. Crab sauce may be made in the same way, using lobster coral if convenient.

No. 31. Bechamel Sauce.—Mix dry in saucepan one tablespoon of flour and two ounces of butter, when well mixed add one pint of milk, dissolve the flour paste, set it on the fire and stir constantly; when it gets thick remove from fire, and add the yolk of one egg well beaten. Add one teaspoon of water, salt and pepper to taste, mix well and it is ready for use. A bouquet of herbs is an improvement to this sauce.

No. 32. Maitre d'Hotel Butter.—Beat four tablespoons of butter to a cream, beating in gradually one tablespoon each of vinegar and lemon juice, half a teaspoon salt, quarter teaspoon pepper, and one teaspoon chopped parsley.

No. 33. Sauce a la Maitre d'Hotel.—Add one teaspoon chopped parsley, juice of one lemon, teaspoon of celery seed, cayenne, and salt to taste to a drawn butter sauce (No. 16.)

No. 34. Sauce Allemande.—Melt two oz. butter and mix thoroughly with two ounces flour over gentle fire; add immediately one pint white stock (No. 14,) a little salt and pepper; stir until boiling, boil fifteen minutes, remove from fire, skim off grease carefully, add yolks of three eggs well mixed in a little water, stir in with egg beater to make sauce light.

No. 35. Sauce a la Aurore.—Coral of one lobster, one oz. butter, half a pint bechamel sauce (No. 31,) juice of half a lemon, liberal seasoning of salt and pepper. Bruise the coral in a mortar with the butter until quite smooth, then rub it through a hair sieve; put the bechamel sauce into stewpan, add the coral paste, lemon juice and seasoning, and let it simmer but not boil— else the red color will be spoiled—pour over the fish, and serve. A small teaspoon of anchovy essence can be added at pleasure. Nice for trout, soles, etc.

No. 36. Blonde Sauce.—To one pint white stock (No. 14) add one sprig parsley, one onion cut into slices, two mushrooms chopped fine, glass of sherry wine, one sliced lemon, put into saucepan and simmer slowly for half an hour, then add yolks of three eggs well whisked and stir over fire for six minutes. Strain through sieve and serve in tureen.

No. 37. Spanish Sauce.—Melt two oz. butter in saucepan, add two oz. flour and stir over gentle fire until a nice brown, mix with this one pint white stock (No. 14,) one and a half oz. lean raw ham, one carrot and one onion sliced, one stalk of celery, two cloves, salt and pepper a pinch each, stir until beginning to boil, then simmer gently on back of range for one hour; skim off grease before serving.

No. 38. White Oyster Sauce.—Put one pint of oysters in a saucepan and let them just come to boiling point, strain and remove the beards; then add to the oyster liquor an equal quantity of milk and a liberal quantity of butter. When hot and smooth add the oysters, heat again without boiling, season and serve in tureen. Thicken with flour smoothed in the milk if desirable.

No. 39. Brown Oyster Sauce.—Proceed same as for white oyster sauce (No. 38,) browning the butter or butter and flour before adding to the milk.

No. 40. Olive Sauce.—Prepare a Maitre d'Hotel butter (No. 32) adding the beaten yolks of two eggs, a little ground mace, and substituting olives for the parsley. Cut the olives in shavings, beginning at one end as you would pare an apple, shaving to the stone and having the shavings thin and whole. Simmer until the olives are tender.

No. 41. Sauce Supreme.—Cut up remains of two roast chickens and put in saucepan with one pint white stock (No. 14,) some branches of parsley enclosing one clove, one clove of garlic, two bay leaves, and a little thyme; tie all together, season with salt and white pepper, boil one hour and strain. Put two oz. butter in another saucepan, and mix with one tablespoon flour and one teaspoon cornstarch; add the strained liquid and stir until boiling, reduce one quarter, put in two wineglasses of cream and one of sherry, boil fifteen minutes more, add juice of one lemon, strain and serve.

No. 42. Celery Sauce.—Cut a head of celery into pieces two inches long, and boil in salted water, enough to cover, in a covered saucepan for one hour. Mix together smoothly, one tablespoon of flour and two of butter, add one pint of milk, and stir until boiling, then strain the celery and add, seasoned with a little salt and pepper and a little powdered mace, let it boil quickly for two minutes, then serve in tureen.

No. 43. Sauce Tartare.—Cold. Chop fine one shallot, with half a tablespoon of chervil, same of tarragon, and twelve capers chopped fine. Put all in an earthen bowl with half a teaspoon of dry mustard, two raw eggs, a teaspoon of vinegar (drop by drop,) salt and pepper. Pour in lightly while stirring, one cup of olive oil, and if too thick add a little more vinegar. Taste until seasoned to suit. Serve with cold salmon.

No. 44. Sauce Tartare.—Hot. One tablespoon vinegar, one teaspoon lemon juice, one saltspoon salt, one tablespoon walnut catsup, two tablespoons butter. Mix vinegar, lemon juice, salt and catsup together and heat over hot water. Brown the butter in another pan, and strain into the other mixture. Nice for broiled fish.

No. 45. Sauce Piquante.—Two ounces butter, one small carrot, six shallots, one small bunch savory herbs, including parsley, half a bay leaf, two slices lean ham, two cloves, six peppercorns, one blade mace, three allspice, four tablespoons vinegar, half a pint stock (No. 14,) half teaspoon sugar, little cayenne, and salt to taste. Put the butter into saucepan with the carrot and shallots cut into small pieces, add the herbs, bay leaf, spices and ham minced fine; let these ingredients simmer slowly until the bottom is covered a brown glaze, keep stirring and put in remaining ingredients, simmer gently fifteen minutes, skim off every particle of fat, strain through sieve and serve very hot, when a sharp but not too acid sauce is required.

No. 46. Sauce Ravigote.—Hot. Put half a pint consomme (No. 14) into saucepan with half a teaspoon vinegar, very little green garlic, same of tarragon leaves and chervil; boil ten minutes, drain herbs and press all moisture from them with a cloth and chop very fine. Put half an ounce flour on the table, same of butter, mix well together and add to the consomme and vinegar, which has been cooking since the herbs were removed, stir until boiling, skim, add chopped herbs and serve. For baked or broiled fish, salmon, Spanish mackerel, bonita and other rich flavored fish.

No. 47. Italian Sauce.—Into a saucepan put half a pint of stock (No. 15) with a few chopped mushrooms and shallots, and a half a glass of Madeira wine. Simmer gently fifteen minutes, then add the juice of half a lemon, half a teaspoon powdered sugar, one teaspoon chopped parsley, and let it come to a boil. Pour over fish and serve.

No. 48. Parisian Sauce.—Put in saucepan half an ounce chopped truffles, wine glass of sherry, some branches parsley, enclosing a clove, a little thyme and a bay leaf, tie all together, reduce one-half, rub through a sieve. Add half a pint sauce allemande (No. 34.) Heat again and serve.

No. 49. Normandy Sauce.—Fry one chopped onion and a few slices of carrot in two tablespoons of butter, thicken with flour, add two tablespoons of Worcestershire sauce, cup of white stock (No. 15) and cup of canned tomatoes, season with pepper and salt. Simmer half an hour, strain and add one dozen chopped mushrooms. Boil five minutes, add one dozen oysters. Boil one minute and pour over fish.

No. 50. Curry Sauce.—Cook one chopped onion in one tablespoon of butter, until slightly browned. Mix one tablespoon of curry powder with two tablespoons of flour. Stir into the butter and onions, adding one pint hot milk gradually, heat and strain.

No. 51. Tomato Sauce.—No. 1. One pound can of tomatoes, two tablespoons of butter, one sliced onion, two tablespoons of flour and a little grated nutmeg. Cook together the tomato, onion and nutmeg for about ten minutes. Heat the butter in a small frying pan and add the flour. Stir until smooth and slightly browned, then stir into the tomatoes. Season to taste, and rub through a strainer fine enough to stop the seeds.

No. 52. Tomato Sauce.—No. 2. Put one oz. lean, raw ham in saucepan with one carrot, one onion, a little thyme, one bay leaf, two cloves, stalk of celery and half oz. of butter. Simmer ten minutes, add one oz. flour well mixed in half a can of tomatoes and three tablespoons of consomme (No. 14.) Boil one hour with salt, pepper and pinch of mace. Strain and serve.

No. 53. Sardine Sauce.—Bone and skin half a dozen sardines, boil the bones and skin in half a pint of stock (No. 15,) or in any fish liquor with a minced shallot, a little lemon peel, a pinch of mace and a little pepper, strain, add the sardines rubbed to a paste, a little butter and cream, sufficient to make of the right consistency. Boil up and serve poured over the fish.

No. 54. Brown Mushroom Sauce.—Peel one dozen mushrooms, chop and fry in butter until a golden brown, then stir into a cream sauce (No. 18,) seasoning to taste.

No. 55. White Mushroom Sauce.—Remove all dark parts, chop and put in saucepan with one gill cream or milk, a small piece of butter and a little white pepper, cover close and simmer very gently until soft, add white stock (No. 14) according to amount of sauce required, a sprinkling of flour having been smoothed into it, let it simmer a few minutes more, with a pinch of mace and a little salt added.

No. 56. Genevese Sauce.—One small carrot, small faggot of sweet herbs, including parsley, one onion, five or six mushrooms, if obtainable, one bay leaf, six cloves, one blade mace, two oz. butter, one glass sherry, one and a half pints white stock (No. 14,) thickening butter and flour, juice of half a lemon. Cut onion and carrot in rings or thin slices and put in saucepan with the herbs, mushrooms, bay leaf, cloves and mace, add the butter and simmer until the onions are quite tender. Pour in the stock and sherry and stir slowly one hour, then strain off into clean saucepan. Now make thickening of butter and flour, put it to the sauce, heat and stir until perfectly smooth, then add lemon juice, give one boil and it is ready to serve with trout or salmon.

No. 57. Fish a la Creme.—After the fish has been dressed and washed, put it into boiling water enough to cover, adding a little salt, pepper and lemon juice; cook slowly about fifteen minutes. Take out the fish and place it on a tray, remove head, bones and skin, preserving its shape as much as possible, only opening it to take out the backbone. Transfer the fish to the platter on which it is to be served, and make a rich cream sauce (No. 18.)

Pour this sauce over the fish and sprinkle the top with bread crumbs, set the platter in a pan of boiling water and bake until the crumbs are brown—say ten minutes.

To prepare the cream, take one quart of milk, or half milk and half cream, two tablespoons of flour, one of butter, one small onion, sliced, a little chopped parsley, salt and pepper; mix half a cup of the milk with the flour, boil the remainder with the onion and parsley, then add the cold milk and flour; cook eight or ten minutes, add the butter, and season highly; strain and pour over the fish as directed. Grated cheese may be added to the crumbs, if liked. The cusk is oftener used for this dish than any other; but it is a good way to serve any of our flavorless fish, as the cod, haddock, pollock, hake, whiting, &c. On the richness of the sauce depends the merit of the dish.

No. 58. Fish a la Creme.—No. 2. Fish weighing four or five pounds, butter size of an egg, three tablespoons of flour, one quart of rich milk, three sprigs of parsley, half an onion, cayenne and salt. Boil the fish in salted water, flake and remove skin and bone. Boil milk, mix butter with flour, stir smooth in the milk, add parsley, chopped fine, chopped onion, cayenne and salt. Butter a dish, put first a layer of fish, then dressing, and continue until dish is full, with dressing on top. Cover with sifted bread crumbs; bake until brown; garnish with parsley.

No. 59. Fish a la Creme.—No. 3. Two pounds fish, one oz. flour, one cup bread crumbs, one quart milk, a little nutmeg, two onions, teaspoon salt, half teaspoon pepper, quarter pound butter. Boil fish and set aside. Put flour into stewpan, add milk gradually, mix smooth, cut onions fine, grate nutmeg, add the salt and pepper, heat and stir until rather thick, add butter, put a layer of this mixture on the serving dish. Flake the fish free from bones and put a layer of this next, then more of the mixture, fish, and so on, until fish is all used. Cover with bread crumbs and bake fifteen or twenty minutes.

No. 60. Fish a la Creme.—No. 4. (Remnants.) Remove skin and bones from cold boiled fish. Boil bones and skin in one pint of milk with a blade of mace and a small onion; strain and thicken with one tablespoon of flour rubbed into an equal quantity of butter; season and let it boil up once. Put as much fish as you have sauce into a deep dish, sprinkle with bread crumbs and bake half an hour.

No. 61. Fish a l' Italienne.—Take one quarter pound of macaroni and break into quite short pieces, put it into hot salted water and boil twenty minutes, drain off the water and stir into the macaroni one tablespoon of butter, three tablespoons grated cheese and one-third as much boiled fish as macaroni, season with salt and pepper, and turn all into a buttered baking dish; wet with milk, scatter bread crumbs on top, bake, covered, for fifteen minutes, then brown and serve. Raw fish may be used, in which case it should bake for thirty minutes before removing cover to brown.

No. 62. Fish a la Maitre d' Hotel.—Take four pounds of fresh cod, or other white-meated fish, and put into boiling salted water and boil for twenty-five minutes, take it up and let it drain, then remove to a hot platter, garnish with parsley and serve with a Maitre d' Hotel sauce (No. 33,) dished separately in tureen.

No. 63. A la Maitre d' Hotel Fish.—Remains of any boiled fish, heat over gentle fire until warmed through; then spread over it a sauce, made by rubbing one tablespoon of butter to a cream, seasoning with pepper, salt, one teaspoon chopped parsley and juice of one lemon. Set it in the oven a moment that butter may penetrate the fish.

No. 64. Fish au Court Bouillon. [1] —This is an improved method of cooking fish in water—by flavoring it with vegetables, spices and acids. To four quarts of water put one quart of good cider vinegar, or a pint of vinegar and the juice of two lemons, and an oz. of salt, or more if needed. Put into a saucepan one chopped onion, two shallots, two stalks of celery, three bay leaves, one sliced carrot and six cloves, with one quart of the water, and simmer all for one hour; strain, and put the sauce in with remainder of prepared water. Rub the fish well with salt, pepper and the juice of a lemon. Let the water boil up once, and skim it before putting in the fish. Boil until flesh separates from the bones. A sauce of drawn butter is the proper accompaniment for fish cooked in this way.

No. 65. Fish au Fromage.—One cup cold boiled macaroni cut into short bits, one cup cold boiled white-meated fish, mixed. Put in buttered dish in alternate layers, with macaroni at the top, season each layer with pepper and salt, moisten with drawn butter, or milk, if more convenient, sprinkle with a few bread crumbs, and over all two tablespoons of grated cheese, bake until brown.

No. 66. Fish au Gratin (baked.)—For this dish use either fillets of fresh fish, or remnants of cooked fish; putting the fish and a bechamel sauce (No. 31) in alternate layers into a deep baking dish and sprinkling crumbs over the top, moistening them with a little melted butter, send to the oven until colored a nice brown.

No. 67. Au Gratin.—Another way is to take three pounds of fillets of fish, season with salt and pepper and lay on a serving dish, sprinkling thickly with sifted cracker crumbs and a little grated Parmesan, or other dry cheese, putting a few bits of butter on top; brown in quick oven and serve at once. A delicate, savory and inexpensive dish.

No. 68. Fish Cake.—Remains of cold cooked fish, one onion, one faggot of sweet herbs, salt and pepper to taste, one pint water, equal quantities bread crumbs and cold potatoes, half a teaspoon parsley, one egg. Flake the fish free from bones and place bones, head and fins in saucepan with the water, add pepper and salt, onion and herbs, and stew slowly about two hours. Chop the fish fine and mix well with bread crumbs and cold potatoes, adding the parsley and seasoning. Make the whole into one cake or several, mixing in the beaten eggs, cover with bread crumbs and fry a light brown in butter. Strain the fish liquor, put the cake in saucepan, pour the liquor over it and stew gently fifteen minutes, stirring once or twice. Serve hot with slices of lemon.

No. 69. Fish a la Vinaigrette.—(Serve cold.) This may be made of fish cooked expressly for the dish, or remnants of almost any kind of cooked fish may be used. The very best fish for the purpose is the striped bass, for its flesh is remarkably white, very firm, and possesses a fine flavor. First stick the fish with cloves, then boil it in vinegar and water. Remove the skin and head, if a whole fish, and set aside to cool. When ready to serve, place it on a napkin on a bed of crisp lettuce. Garnish with sprigs of parsley, slices of cucumber, water cresses, sliced lemon, or boiled sliced beats, any of these are suitable. Serve with a sauce tartare (No. 43.) If remnants of cooked fish are used, they should be heaped in the center of the dish and garnished same as the whole fish, and the sauces may be served separately, or poured over the fish; if the latter way, it should not be garnished until the same is poured over it. A nice hot weather dish.

No. 70. Fish Cakes.—Mix together, cold, cooked fish, mashed potatoes, butter, seasoning and the yolk of a well beaten egg, and if necessary moisten with milk or cream, shape into round flat cakes, dip them in beaten egg, roll in crumbs and fry a light brown, drain and serve on a napkin. A very nice way to use remnants of cooked fish. A teaspoon of chopped parsley is an improvement.

No. 71. Fish and Oyster Cakes.—Substitute oysters for the potato in No. 70, having equal quantities of fish and oysters, and mixing in crumbs enough to make the mixture hold together.

No. 72. Casserole of Fish.—Flake free from bones and skin one pint cooked fish; mix with it, one cup of stale bread crumbs and two beaten eggs. Season with salt and pepper, add a pinch of mace, a teaspoon of Worcestershire sauce and a few drops of lemon juice. Boil in buttered mould and serve with oyster sauce (No. 38.)

No. 73. Chartreuse of Fish.—Flake and season one cup cold, cooked fish, moisten with a little cream or milk. Use an equal quantity of mashed potato and two hard boiled eggs in slices. Butter a small mould and put in alternate layers of potato, fish and sliced eggs. Season with salt, pepper, onion juice and a speck of cayenne. Steam twenty minutes, turn out on platter and garnish with parsley. Serve with, or without a sauce poured over or separately.

No. 74. Fish Chowder.—No fish chowder should have bones in it; to avoid this, dress, wash and cut up your fish and put it on to boil in cold water, without salt; as soon as it is cooked enough—say ten minutes—for the flesh to be separated from the bones, take it up and remove all bones; put the head, bones, etc., back into the water, and boil until water is wanted. In the meantime you should fry in the bottom of your chowder kettle some small dice-shaped pieces of salt pork, say one quarter pound of pork for every five pounds of fish; when the pork is all tried out and nicely browned, but not burnt, put in some thinly sliced onions in quantity to suit, and cook these until yellow, not brown; now put in one quart of cold water (for five pounds of fish,) strain the bone water and put that in, then some sliced potatoes, season with salt and pepper, and when the potatoes are nearly done put in the fish; boil one quart of milk and add to the chowder; now try it and see if it is seasoned all right; let all come to a boil, pour into a tureen and serve. A common way is to put a layer of crackers on top of the chowder when the milk is put in; but many prefer the crackers served separately. Clam water added to a fish chowder is a great improvement.

No. 75. St. James Fish Chowder.—Put half pound sliced salt pork in bottom of kettle and fry brown, then remove the pork and put in layers of potatoes, onions and fish sliced, seasoning each layer with salt and pepper. Use one quart each, potatoes and onions to three pounds of fish, cover with cold water and bring to a boil gradually and cook slowly for half an hour, then add two pounds sea biscuit soaked for five minutes in warm water, boil five minutes more and serve immediately after adding half a pint of port wine and a bottle of champagne. Milk may be substituted for the wine and it will be quite good enough and far less expensive.

No. 76. Major Henshaws Fish Chowder.—Cut up one and a half, or two pounds, salt pork and put in kettle, covering close, when nearly tried out remove the pieces of pork and put in four tablespoons sliced onions, when browned slightly, put in six pounds fish in slices, one and a half pounds broken crackers, twenty-five large oysters, one quart mashed, boiled potatoes, half a dozen large tomatoes sliced (or an equal quantity tomato catsup,) one bottle port wine or claret, half a grated nutmeg, teaspoon each, summer savory and thyme, a few cloves, blade of mace, allspice, black pepper and slices lemon. Put fish, crackers, etc., all in layers in the order stated, sprinkling in the other ingredients, add water enough to cover and simmer, not boil, until fish on top is done. This chowder too is good enough for a king without the wine.

No. 77. Creamed Fish.—Scald two cups of milk, when hot, stir in one tablespoon butter, braided with one teaspoon flour, when it thickens remove from fire; butter pudding dish and fill with layers of cooked fish, season with salt and pepper and wet with the thickened milk. Sprinkle over the top a few fine cracker crumbs. Bake about twenty minutes.

No. 78. Creamed Fish with Oysters.—Use the same quantity of oysters as of boneless cooked fish and cook in a cream sauce until the oysters are plump.

No. 79. Crimped Fish.—Cut uncooked fish in long thin strips, roll them around the finger and fasten each roll or crimp with a wooden toothpick. Soak half an hour in strong salted water, then put into boiling salted water, enough to cover, with two tablespoons vinegar and boil about fifteen minutes. Drain, arrange on a platter, removing skin and bones, and serve hot with oyster or lobster sauce poured into cavities made by the finger.

No. 80. Crumbed Fish.—Remove bones and skin from cold, boiled, white-meated fish and pick into flakes. Boil bones with one onion. Season the fish with salt and pepper and fill the buttered baking dish half full. Pour in remains of drawn butter, or prepare a little for the purpose, sprinkle with bread crumbs, add the remainder of the fish, put in more crumbs, moisten with the water in which bones were boiled, bake about twenty minutes. Should be more moist than scalloped oysters.

No. 81. Fish Croquettes.—One pint of cold, boiled fish minced fine, free from bones and skin. Bring half a pint of milk to a boil, thicken with two tablespoons of flour rubbed smooth, with a tablespoon of butter. Remove from fire, add the fish, season with teaspoon of chopped parsley, pepper and salt. When the mixture gets cold, form into oval shaped balls, dip in egg or cracker crumbs and fry in hot fat.

No. 82. Curried Fish.—Put two oz. of butter and one sliced onion into frying pan and cook until a delicate brown, then add one tablespoon of flour mixed in a cup of water in which fish was boiled, one cup of cream, or milk and one teaspoon curry powder. Remove all bones from fish, taking care not to break it into small pieces. Stir the sauce until it boils, then add fish, cover and set the dish into another of hot water, cook half an hour, serve with steamed or boiled rice.

No. 83. Fish Dressing.—(For a small fish.) Two tablespoons bread crumbs, a desertspoon of parsley after it is washed, dried in a cloth and chopped fine, a little thyme and marjoram, discarding the stalks. Mix herbs and crumbs together, add pepper and salt and two oz. suet chopped fine.

No. 84. Fish Dressing.—(For a fish of five pounds.) Chop fine one pint of oysters, add to them half pint rolled cracker crumbs, one tablespoon of butter, quarter teaspoon of pepper, half teaspoon each, salt and celery salt and one of chopped parsley. Mix all together thoroughly, moistening with milk if necessary and adding a few drops onion juice.

No. 85. Fish Dressing.—(For a fish of five pounds.) Half a pound of dry, stale bread, two beaten eggs, teaspoon salt, half teaspoon pepper, few drops onion juice, one teaspoon each powdered marjoram, summer savory and parsley, two tablespoons butter. Moisten the bread first with boiling water, then add eggs, butter, seasoning and herbs and mix well together, moistening with milk as needed.

No. 86. Fish Dressings.—(For a fish of five pounds.) Mash one pint hot, boiled potatoes and two boiled onions together, season with salt, pepper and chopped parsley, moisten with butter and milk.

Fish Dressing.—(For a fish of six pounds.) Roll fine six butter crackers and add to them half a teaspoon chopped parsley, one tablespoon chopped salt pork, salt and pepper to taste, mix well, moistening with cold water or milk.

No. 87. Farce.—Place in a saucepan four oz. very fresh bread crumbs and one cup consomme (No. 14,) simmer gently ten minutes, at the end of which time stir constantly with a wooden spoon and boil ten minutes longer so as to form a stiff paste. This done put it on a plate to cool. Take four oz. breast of chicken from which remove the skin and sinews and pound extremely fine, add to this the bread crumbs in quantity about three quarters as much as there is of the chicken and pound together until well mixed, season with a little salt and pepper, a very little nutmeg and a piece of butter; then pound again adding by degrees two eggs, until you have obtained a fine, smooth paste. Small, delicate fish, like trout, may be stuffed with this farce, or it may be made into quenelles by forming into small balls and poaching for two minutes in boiling water. Serve in fish soups and with baked or boiled fish.

No. 88. Fish en Vinaigrette.—Boil the fish, which may be bass or halibut, in salt water for ten minutes to each pound. When done, stand it aside to cool. When cold, place it in the centre of a large dish. Chop fine the whites and yolks of two hard-boiled eggs, but keep them separate; also chop sufficient parsley to make two tablespoonfuls. Put a string of the yolks next to the fish; next to this put a string of whites, next capers and sprinkle the whole with chopped parsley. Split a lemon in two lengths; then each half into four pieces, and place these on each side of the fish, or the fish may simply be served on a bed of lettuce with a sauce tartare (No. 43.)

No. 89. Forcemeat.—Two oz. lean ham, or bacon, quarter pound suet, peel of half a lemon, one teaspoon minced parsley, teaspoon minced sweet herbs, salt, cayenne and mace to taste, six oz. bread crumbs, two eggs. Shred the ham, or bacon, chop the suet, the lemon peel and mix all together with the minced herbs, seasoning and bread crumbs before wetting. Then beat and strain the eggs and work them in with the other ingredients and the forcemeat is ready for use. When made into balls it may be fried, or baked on a tin in the oven half an hour. No one flavor should predominate greatly, and the forcemeat should be sufficiently firm to cut with a knife, but not dry and heavy.

No. 90. Forcemeat.—Meat of one boiled lobster, half a sardine, one head boiled celery, yolk of one hard-boiled egg, salt, cayenne and mace to taste, four tablespoons bread crumbs, two oz. butter, two eggs. Pound the lobster meat and the soft parts in a mortar, add the celery, egg yolk, seasoning and bread crumbs and continue until the whole is nicely mixed. Melt the butter a little, beat up the eggs and work into the pounded lobster meat. Make into balls about an inch in diameter and fry of a nice pale brown. Serve with any fish that cannot be stuffed.

No. 91. Fricassee au Gratin.—Take two pounds of fish, free from bones and skin and cut in small pieces. Mix together half a pint of cream, one tablespoon of anchovy sauce, one tablespoon of tomato ketchup, a little salt and pepper; thicken with flour and butter rubbed smooth, heat very hot and put into the serving dish, lay in the fish, strew with cracker or bread crumbs and a few bits of butter, bake and brown.

No. 92. Golden Fillets.—Cut your fish into fillets, trimming away all ragged edges, then lay them for fifteen minutes in a mixture prepared as follows: One tablespoon of salad oil, one teaspoon of Chili vinegar, one of tarragon vinegar, one each of parsley and onion, chopped fine, a scant saltspoon of salt and one quarter as much pepper, mixed together smoothly. Take out the fillets and drain them, then dip each fillet into a batter made with one tablespoon of milk mixed with two oz. of flour and one tablespoon of oil to a smooth paste, then add yolks of two eggs and the whites whipped fine with one quarter saltspoon of salt. Fry each fillet separately in a wire basket three minutes in very hot fat. Drain and serve on a napkin.

No. 93. Kromeskies of Fish.—Prepare the fish as for croquettes; form into small rolls, and envelope each in a slice of salt pork, cut as thin as possible; fasten in place by the use of small wooden toothpicks. Dip in beaten egg, roll in crumbs, and fry in hot fat.

No. 94. Kedgeree.—Flake remnants of cooked fish, free from bones and skin, add hard-boiled egg chopped, and a cup of steamed rice. Mix all well together, with cream or butter to moisten, adding a little cayenne, salt and mustard. Put all into a saucepan and stir with a fork, until quite hot.

No. 95. Marinade of Fish.—Hot. Prepare the fish for stewing, pour over it a marinade and simmer until done. To make the *Marinade* take a sliced onion, a few slices of carrot and cook in two tablespoons of butter, with one teaspoon salt and simmer for ten minutes, then add one quart of cider, half a teaspoon pepper and the same of mustard, four cloves and a bouquet of sweet herbs. Cover and simmer one and a half hours. Strain and pour over the fish and stew.

No. 96. Marinade.—Cold. Bouquet sweet herbs, juice of half a lemon, two tablespoons of oil, six of vinegar, one teaspoon onion juice, cayenne, teaspoon salt, one quarter teaspoon pepper, little ground clove. Mix all together and sprinkle over any fish prepared for broiling, and let it stand five or six hours before cooking.

No. 97. Matelote of Fish.—Take fillets of any white-meated fish and soak for an hour in port wine; then put them in a saucepan with a bouquet of herbs, a cup of stock, a glass of wine, chopped onions, parsley, mushrooms, salt and pepper, simmer half an hour. Dish the fish, strain the gravy, add half a pint of cream, heat and pour over fish; squeeze in the juice of a lemon, and serve hot.

No. 98. Mariners Matelote of Fish.—Take any live fish, dress but do not wash, (for mariners hold, a fish once out of water should never go back to it.) Cut in small pieces without losing the blood. Put all into stewpan with a couple dozen small white onions, scalded and almost cooked. Season with salt, pepper, bay leaf and lemon peel, add enough claret or red vin ordinaire to cover the fish. Boil over a quick fire, but do not let the wine ignite, put in a lump of butter size of walnut, arrange the fish on slices of toast and pour the sauce over it. We recommend, however, that the fish be dressed and cleaned.

No. 99. Fish Collops.—Cut two pounds of fish into small pieces, put bones and trimmings, with a small onion chopped, a tablespoon of butter, pepper, salt and mace in saucepan and make a broth, strain and thicken it. Fry the collops brown, and then stew them gently in the broth fifteen minutes. After dishing them add one teaspoon of walnut catsup and a teaspoon of lemon juice to the gravy, pour over the collops and serve hot, garnish with slices of lemon.

No. 100. Minced Fish.—To three cups flaked boiled fish add one cup mashed potato, piece of butter size of a filbert, half teaspoon cornstarch and one beaten egg; heat all together with seasoning, salt and pepper, adding eggs last.

No. 101. Fish Omelet.—Take a cup of cooked fish, remove all bones and skin, chop rather coarse, season with salt and pepper and warm up in cream, butter or milk, whichever is most convenient. Make a plain omelet with six eggs; when ready to fold spread on the hot fish, roll up and serve hot.

No. 102. Fish and Oyster Omelet.—Use half a cup of cooked fish free from bones and skin, add to it a half cup of oysters, season and warm up together in cream and proceed as in fish omelet (No. 101;) serve hot.

No. 103. Fish Pie.—Remains of cooked fish, one dozen oysters, melted butter to moisten. Flake the fish free from bones and skin, put in pie dish, pour over it the melted butter and oysters, cover with mashed potato. Bake half an hour browning nicely.

No. 104. Fish Pie.—Take the remains of any cooked fish, white-meated being preferable, remove bones, skin, etc., season with pepper, salt and mace. To each pound of fish add one dozen oysters. Put a layer of fish in the baking dish, then oysters, then more fish, and so on to the top. Pour in half a cup of stock or water, put bits of butter on top, cover with puff paste and bake half an hour. Make a cream sauce and pour into the pie before serving.

No. 105. Pickled Fish.—Boil four pounds of fish until the bones can be picked out, when cold cut into slices an inch thick; take vinegar enough to cover the fish, add a dozen cloves, a dozen peppercorns, one teaspoon mace, one of allspice, one of celery seed and one of salt; boil ten minutes, pour over the fish, cover close and serve cold.

No. 106. Potted Fish.—Shad, mackerel, alewives, herrings, or smelts may be used in potting, the fatter they are the better. Prepare the fish as for frying, removing heads and tails but saving roes. Cut the fish into pieces one inch long and put them with the roes, in stone jars in layers, packing closely, and putting seasoning and spices between the layers. For six pounds of fish use half a cup mixed whole spices, one chopped onion (if the flavor is not objectionable,) one teaspoon celery salt, one teaspoon table salt and one dozen peppercorns. On top put one bay leaf and one blade of mace, adding vinegar enough to cover. Cover the jar tightly with paper and bake in moderate oven five or six hours. Will keep some time, if kept covered with vinegar and the jar covered closely. Very nice for lunch in hot weather. The flavor and seasoning may be varied to suit individual tastes and convenience.

No. 107. Fish Pyramid.—Flake with a fork two cups cold boiled white-meated fish and put in saucepan with drawn butter, season with salt and pepper and add one cup boiled rice, sprinkle in one teaspoon curry powder, when all is well heated pile on hot platter, garnish with sliced hard boiled eggs and a little chopped parsley.

No. 108. Rissoles of Cooked Fish.—Any remnants of cooked fish may be used, but white-meated fish are preferable. Remove all bones, and pick fine. Mix with an equal quantity of bread crumbs and a little butter, add an onion chopped fine, a little chopped parsley, sprinkling of sage, and season with salt and pepper, mixing in beaten egg enough to make it hold together. Make into small flat cakes, and fry in hot butter. When done, add a little water to the fat in pan, dredge in a little flour, stir in a tablespoon of chopped capers, pour round the rissoles, and serve hot.

No. 109. Fish Roes.—Roes and spawns are but different names given to the eggs found in the female fish. The male has a roe, usually called the milt, but it is doubtful if it has any edible value, though in some of the recipes of old times we find it is occasionally utilized in the making of sauces, dressing, etc. The roe of the shad is now esteemed a delicacy, though formerly considered of little value. The haddock roe ranks next in commercial importance, but we believe there are others superior to it if not equal to those of the shad. Nearly all are eatable when in condition and that of the striped bass is a favorite with foreigners. As a rule the roe is in best condition when the fish is most desirable for the table. The shad is best in the spring, the time varying with the location when caught. Only the roe of a perfectly fresh fish is really good. Fish roes should be handled carefully to keep from breaking. Soak in salted water for a few minutes before cooking, always wiping dry, if large they should be parboiled before frying, and then if very large split in two after parboiling.

No. 110. Fish Roes to Fry.—This is the usual method of cooking, dipping the roes in beaten egg and rolling in crumbs. They should be well done, and require considerable cooking. Unless perfectly dry when put into the hot fat it will sputter badly. Drain each roe on paper when taken up. Serve hot on a napkin garnished with sprigs of parsley.

No. 111. Scalloped Fish Roes.—Wash in salted water, wipe dry and cook ten minutes in boiling salted water, with one tablespoon of vinegar, then plunge them into cold water, drain and break into small particles with a fork and sprinkle into shallow dish in layers, between which sprinkle the yolks of hard-boiled eggs pulverized, a little chopped parsley and a few drops lemon juice, moisten the whole with a thin white, or cream sauce (No. 18,) season, cover with buttered crumbs and bake until brown.

No. 112. Fish Roe Croquettes.—For one pair of good sized roes take half a pint cream, two tablespoons cornstarch, two tablespoons butter, one-half teaspoon salt, juice of one lemon, a little ground mace and a speck of cayenne. Boil the roes in salted water and one teaspoon lemon juice for fifteen minutes, then drain and mash. Boil the cream and stir into it while boiling the butter and cornstarch well smoothed together, add seasoning and roe, boil up once and set away to cool. Shape in croquettes when cold, dip in beaten egg, roll in crumbs and fry in hot fat, drain and serve hot on a napkin, garnished with sliced cucumbers.

No. 113. Fish Roes a la Creole.—Boil two large roes in salted water with one tablespoon vinegar, two cloves, a blade of mace, a little lemon peel, three peppercorns and three whole allspice for fifteen minutes, then drain, wipe dry and fry in butter, browning both sides. Serve with one cup stewed tomatoes poured over them, or with beefsteak tomato ketchup.

No. 114. Scalloped Fish.—Remnants of cold cooked fish, picked free from bones, skin, etc., half a pint of cream, half a tablespoon of anchovy sauce, half a teaspoon of made mustard, same of walnut ketchup, seasoning with pepper and salt. Put all ingredients into stewpan, heat hot, but do not boil. When done put into deep scallop dish and cover with bread crumbs and bits of butter. Set in the oven to brown.

No. 115. Scalloped Fish.—Take remnants of cold, boiled fish, remove bones, skin, etc., and reduce to flakes. Make a sauce with equal quantities of milk and cream, stirring flour into the cold milk and adding it to the boiling cream. Cook five or six minutes, season well, and put a layer of the sauce into bottom of baking dish, then a layer of fish, and so on to the top; season each layer and cover all with bread crumbs. Bake half an hour.

No. 116. Fish Scalloped.—Mix together two cups mashed potato, one and a half cups cold boiled fish, two cups milk, one egg, and one-quarter cup of butter; put in pudding dish and bake a light brown.

No. 117. Fish Scalloped with Macaroni.—Butter earthen pudding dish and place in it coarse flakes of boiled fish and add an equal quantity of cooked macaroni. Pour over it a cream sauce (No. 18) well seasoned with pepper and salt and a little mace, grate cheese on top or use bread crumbs if preferred, dot with bits of butter and bake about twenty minutes.

No. 118. Fish Scallops.—Remains of any cold, cooked white-meated fish; to each half pound fish add half a cup stewed tomatoes, half tablespoon anchovy sauce, half teaspoon made mustard, same of walnut ketchup, pepper, salt and bread crumbs. Pick fish free of bones and put into saucepan with all the other ingredients, heat without boiling, stirring the while. Take out the fish and put into scallop shells, sprinkle freely with bread crumbs, put bits of butter on top, brown and serve.

No. 119. Fish Scallops.—Add one cup soft clams chopped, to No. 114, and cook in shells.

No. 120. Fish Scallops.—Remnants of cooked fish, one egg, wine glass of wine, one blade pounded mace, one tablespoon flour, one tablespoon tomato ketchup, pepper, salt, bread crumbs, butter. Pick the fish from bones and skin, moisten with wine and beaten egg, add the other ingredients, put in scallop shells, cover with bread crumbs, dot with bits of butter, brown and serve.

No. 121. Fish Souffle.—Take one cup cold, baked fish and mix gradually with one cup of mashed potato, season with salt and pepper, stir in one well beaten egg, put in buttered dish and set in oven until very hot, beat the white and yolk of another egg separately, beating the white very stiff, add pepper and salt to the yolk, stir in the white, heap over the fish and put in the oven to brown.

No. 122. Fish Soup.—Boil two pounds fish in two quarts salted water, with a small onion, until it is all boiled to pieces; then rub it through a sieve, add one quart of milk, a tablespoon of butter, a little chopped parsley, salt and pepper to taste. Boil up again and serve.

No. 123. Hustled Clams.—This is the plainest way of serving the long clam and although a very inelegant dish is a most palatable one, especially at the seaside and in the camp. To a peck of clams, after washing thoroughly, add one gill of water, cover close and boil until those on top are well opened, then pour the contents of the kettle, water and all, into a large pan and put it in the centre of the table. Serve to each person plain melted butter, to which let each add, to suit, vinegar and pepper. Take the clams in the fingers, remove from the shell, pull off the black skin that covers the snout and runs around the clam, then take the clam with the thumb and finger by the snout, dip him in the butter, and eat all but the black snout, which you will bite off. Brownbread is a very appropriate accompaniment, and is usually served with baked clams at the famous clam bakes, where the process of eating is the same.

No. 124. Clam Soup.—For clam soups, or chowders, it is better to open the clams raw, but if too much trouble, boil them enough to open the shells; in either case save the liquor to put in the soup. In what ever way clams are to be cooked or eaten, the black skin that covers the snout and surrounds the clam must be discarded, as well as the black part of the snout itself. Unless the clams are very small it is better to chop the hard parts before putting into soups or chowders, the soft part may be used whole. To make the soup, take the liquor from one quart of clams and put in double boiler with an equal quantity of water, season with pepper and mace and salt if needed; boil five minutes, put in the clams, cover close, and boil from five to fifteen minutes; the difference depending upon whether the clams have already been partially cooked; add one pint of boiling milk, or more to suit, thickened a little with flour and butter, or fine cracker dust; butter some split crackers and lay in bottom of tureen and pour the soup over them. This may be varied in many ways and the quantity of milk used must depend upon the amount of clam liquor available. Chopped celery, or onion, or both, improves the flavor for some people, and some like a teaspoon of chopped parsley.

No. 125. Clam Chowder.—There are innumerable ways of making this chowder, every cook book has one or more recipes for it, yet, hardly any two are alike. We give recipes for two ways of making, which we do not think can be improved upon. For the first one open clams enough to make a quart without the liquor, which you save and strain for the chowder. Cut a quarter pound of salt pork into small dice shape pieces, put it into the bottom of the kettle and fry brown, without burning, adding, at the same time, four sliced onions, or more, to suit; keep stirring until the pork is all tried out and the onions slightly colored. Then add the clam water and an equal quantity of fresh water, when it boils, add six good sized potatoes, sliced very thin, or chopped, cover close and cook until the potatoes are done, have ready one quart boiling milk and add with clams, season with pepper, cover and cook, until the clams are done, pour into tureen and serve.

No. 126. Clam Chowder No. 2.—Take the same quantity of clams as for the previous chowder and prepare as for clam soup. Put a layer of clams in the bottom of kettle then a layer of hard crackers, split, buttered and peppered, then more clams and crackers until the clams are all used, the top layer being crackers; add clam liquor and water enough to cover, cook slowly at first, then let it boil briskly fifteen minutes if the clams are raw. Have ready a pint of boiling milk, add to the chowder, boil up once. Sliced onions can be used in this chowder, but should be boiled until nearly done before adding them. Place some of them on each layer of clams. Sliced tomatoes may be used instead of the crackers. Season to taste.

No. 127. Clams a la Creme.—Chop boiled clams, but not very fine. For one quart melt two tablespoons of butter and thicken smooth with the same quantity of flour, season with pepper and a speck of mace or nutmeg and add the clams, simmer three minutes and add one cup boiling cream. If the cream is not boiled before adding it is liable to curdle. A little clam water may be added, also. Arrange split and buttered crackers on a hot platter and pour the creamed clams over them.

No. 128. Steamed Clams.—Steamed clams are preferred to either boiled or baked by some people. Wash the clams clean, and pack them into a steamer edgewise so the water will all drain off when they cook, cover closely and steam until the shells open well. Serve the clams in the half shells after removing black skin and cutting off the black end; scissors are better than a knife for this purpose. Serve melted butter and brownbread with steamed clams. If it is desirable to save the clam water, put the clams into the kettle without any water.

No. 129. Clam Water.—Whenever clam water is wanted for any purpose in cooking it should be put into a pitcher and allowed to stand until well settled, then pour off carefully, if drained through a sieve the small particles of sand are liable to go through even the finest of sieves.

No. 130. Bisque of Clams.—Boil one quart of small clams out of the shell in their own liquor for five minutes, then drain. Put in saucepan, four oz. butter, with two oz. flour, heat smooth and add the clams and their liquor, a little salt, pepper and a speck of cayenne, then stir in one quart boiling milk, boil up and serve.

No. 131. Purce of Clams.—A purce of clams or other shell fish is made the same as for a bisque, except that the clams are rubbed through a sieve forming a soft paste before adding the milk.

No. 132. Scalloped Clams.—Clams may be scalloped same as oysters, but only the soft parts should be used and those should be boiled in the shell just enough so they can be opened easily. Some of the clam liquor should be used to moisten the cracker crumbs.

No. 133. Clam Croquettes.—Chop the boiled clams and mix with cracker crumbs, moistening with clam liquor and cream, seasoning to taste, form into croquettes and fry in hot fat, or the clams may be bruised to a paste. Drain the croquettes on paper, or a sieve, and serve on a napkin.

No. 134. Clams au Gratin.—Chop the hard parts and mix with the soft. To a cup of clams add a cup of bread or cracker crumbs, add also one teaspoon of finely chopped onion, half a teaspoon of powdered marjoram and sage, the same of chopped celery, a little cayenne and salt if needed. Moisten with clam liquor and boiled cream, put into baking dish, sprinkle crumbs over the top, dot with bits of butter and bake a nice brown.

No. 135. Clams a la Creole.—Prepare same as for au gratin and moisten with canned tomatoes instead of the cream and clam liquor. For either this dish, or clams au gratin, if only the soft parts of the clams are used they will be found much nicer.

No. 136. Clams on Toast.—Open raw, chop the hard parts and mix with the soft, warm them up in their own liquor, with butter, seasoning and a dash of bruised mace. Have toast ready, either bread or crackers, well buttered, strain the liquor over the toast, then spread on the clams. Serve hot. Cream, or wine, or both, added to the liquor will be found an improvement.

No. 137. Fried Clams.—Select good, plump clams, dry them on a towel, roll in cracker crumbs, dip in egg, again in crumbs, and fry in hot fat; lay a sheet of paper in a colander and put the clams on this as fast as taken up; serve them on a napkin on a hot platter. The paper will prevent them from being greasy when sent to the table.

No. 138. Scalloped Clams.—For this prepare 25 clams, one-half pint cracker crumbs, one-half cup warm milk, one-fourth cup of clam liquor, two beaten eggs, one heaping teaspoonful melted butter, salt and pepper, 12 clam shells; season the clams highly; mix in another dish crackers moistened first with milk, then with the clam liquor; add eggs and melted butter, and the clams chopped; fill each clam shell heaping, sprinkle with bread crumbs and brown.

No. 139. Clam Fritters.—Either whole clams or chopped may be used. Prepare a good batter, stir in the clams, using considerable clam liquor in making the batter. If whole clams are used the large ones are the best, having one in each fritter; when the chopped clams are used the fritters may be made any size to suit. Drain and serve on a napkin. Parboil the clams before opening.

No. 140. Soft Clams Stewed.—Soft clams, so called, are merely the soft parts used without any of the hard parts (there are no other soft clams.) To stew them put the soft parts, raw, into saucepan with a little butter, simmer a few minutes and add boiling cream, with half as much clam water, season with salt and cayenne, add a little cracker dust, simmer three minutes longer and serve. As the clam water is always used to increase the clam flavor, more or less may be used to suit the taste.

No. 141. Quahogs or Round Clams.—These require very much more cooking than the long clam. Quahog shells, as well as those of the sea clam, are very useful for all kinds of shell fish scallops and it is a good plan to keep them on hand for this purpose.

No. 142. Quahogs Raw.—These are highly esteemed by some people, the medium size, or even quite small ones, being preferable; they should be served on the half shell, with vinegar, or lemon juice and pepper, or with Worcestershire sauce.

No. 143. Quahog Cocktail.—This is in great favor at some of the New York cafés, though it is usually called a "clam cocktail." Take six of the tiniest quahogs obtainable and put them in a glass with a tablespoon of the clam liquor, add a speck of cayenne, a saltspoon of ground celery, a teaspoon of tomato catsup, a teaspoon of vinegar and one of Worcestershire sauce. Stir thoroughly with a fork and eat one by one. When the clams are gone, drink the remaining contents of the glass. Those who know, say this is delicious beyond comparison.

No. 144. Quahogs a la Provincetown.—If you want to eat clams of any kind served to perfection go to Cape Cod. Many people dislike the quahog because they cannot cook it tender, but they serve up a quahog stew in Provincetown with the quahogs as tender as a chicken. The quahogs are opened raw, and with their liquor and some water besides, are put on to cook immediately after breakfast and at noontime they are tender enough for anybody. After coming to a boil they should merely simmer until half an hour before serving, when sliced potatoes are added and they are allowed to cook faster until these are done. No more liquid should be used than just enough to keep the stew from sticking; the only seasoning used is pepper. Ten minutes before taking up cover the top of the stew with buttered crackers split in two. Pour the entire contents of kettle on to a platter and serve. The long clam is also very good stewed in this way, but the clams do not need to stew more than half an hour before the potatoes are put in. Try it and be convinced.

No. 145. Quahog Chowder.—This is made the same as the clam chowder, only the quahogs must be chopped very fine, and must be put in at the same time the potatoes are put in. Quahogs may also be cooked in any way that the long clam is cooked, remembering that they must either be chopped very fine, or be allowed more time in cooking.

No. 146. Mussel Chowder.—The mussels that are found so plenty on some of our beaches make a very nice *chowder*. Select those that are fresh always, and these can be easily distinguished by the shells being tightly closed; if the shells are open and remain so the mussel is not fit to eat. Parboil them in the shell, then open and remove the black, mossy substance, the rest is eatable. Cook the same as the long clam, they are very tender and require but little cooking.

No. 147. Scallops.—The shell of the scallop is round and deeply grooved on both sides.—from whence it takes its name probably. The eatable part is the muscle which unites the shell. The dark colored rim should be discarded. The scallop has a sweet flavor and is so rich, however cooked, that the appetite is soon cloyed. Scallops can be stewed the same as oysters, or fried in batter, or crumbs.

No. 148. Scalloped Scallops.—This is a delicious dish. Take the scallops out raw, discard the dark rim, cut the scallops into small pieces and mix with cracker crumbs, beaten egg and a little milk or cream, seasoning to taste. Fill some of the shells, washed for the purpose, cover with crumbs, put a bit of butter on each and bake a delicate brown.

No. 149. Scallop Fritters, or Fried in Crumbs.—No shell fish can surpass the scallop. Fried in crumbs, or fried in batter, it is fully equal to the oyster.

No. 150. Seaside Scallop.—This is a great delicacy, and composed of equal proportions of chopped lobster, crab, oyster, clam and scallops. Mix all together with cracker crumbs and beaten egg, seasoning to taste, adding a little chopped celery, chopped mushrooms and parsley. Moisten with cream and sherry wine equally; fill clam shells; sprinkle crumbs on top, with bits of butter; bake a delicate brown and serve hot.

No. 151. Crabs.—There are three varieties of crabs, all of which are highly prized by the epicure. The large, blue crab is eaten both hard and soft shell, but the latter is esteemed the greater delicacy. Oyster crabs have lately taken their place among luncheon dainties. These are all in the markets the year round.

No. 152. Boiled Crabs.—Hard-shell crabs require about fifteen minutes to boil, and may be served plain, same as boiled lobster, either hot or cold, all but the spongy substance being eatable, but the better way is to pick out the meat and serve by some of the following recipes:

No. 153. Soft-Shell Crabs to Cook.—These are either fried or broiled whole. To prepare them for cooking, lift the shell at both edges and remove the gray, spongy substance, which can be plainly seen, then pull off the little triangular apron like piece on under side of shell, wash and wipe the crabs dry, dip in milk and roll in flour and fry in hot fat, five minutes ought to suffice; or dip in beaten egg and roll in crumbs, and either fry or broil.

No. 154. Scalloped Crabs.—No. 1. To one pint boiled crab meat, picked fine, add a little nutmeg, or mace, one tablespoon cracker or bread crumbs, two eggs well beaten and two tablespoons butter; mix well, and fill the crab shells, cleaned for the purpose, put crumbs on top and a bit of butter for each and put in the oven to brown.

No. 155. Scalloped Crabs.—No. 2. Pick fine one pint boiled crab meat and mix with a cream sauce (No. 18,) salt and pepper, fill the crab shells, cover with buttered cracker crumbs and bake brown.

No. 156. Devilled Crabs.—Mix one pint chopped crab meat with the yolks of two hard boiled eggs, chopped, one tablespoon of bread crumbs, juice of half a lemon, half a teaspoon prepared mustard, a little cayenne, salt and one cup drawn butter. When well mixed, fill the crab shells, sprinkle crumbs over the top, heat slightly and brown in quick oven.

No. 157. Crabs a la Creole.—Put into saucepan, one oz. of butter, one onion chopped fine, and a little water, season with salt, cayenne and mace; simmer for fifteen minutes, add half a pint strained tomato pulp, a gill of chicken broth and a little celery salt. Cut six soft-shelled crabs in halves, removing the spongy parts and put them into the sauce; simmer eight minutes and serve.

No. 158. Farcied Crabs.—Remove meat from four dozen boiled, hard-shell crabs and chop fine. Put in a saucepan one chopped onion and one oz. butter, when beginning to color slightly add one dozen chopped mushrooms and four oz. bread crumbs, which have been previously soaked in consomme (No. 14) and then press nearly dry, add salt, pepper, cayenne and half a gill tomato ketchup. Mix all well together while heating and cook five minutes. Clean the crab shells, fill with the mixture, cover with crumbs and a little butter, brown in oven a light color. Lobster may be served in the same way.

No. 159. Crab Saute.—Soft-shell crabs cut in two and all objectionable matter removed may be sauted in butter or salad oil, with a seasoning to suit. Canned crab meat may be served in the same way.

No. 160. Crab Toast.—Put one pint boiled crab meat in saucepan, with melted butter, one teaspoon chopped celery, a pinch of flour, a gill of cream, salt and pepper to taste; simmer until reduced to suitable consistency for spreading on thin slices of toast; garnish with a few oyster crabs on each slice. A dash of sherry is an improvement. Lobster toast may be made in same way.

No. 161. Crab Bisque.—Boil four hard-shelled crabs in salted water for fifteen minutes, wash and drain and pound in a mortar; add one quart of white broth, one bouquet of herbs, tablespoon of rice, salt and pepper and boil three-quarters of an hour; strain through a fine sieve, add one cup of cream, heat without boiling, and serve with small squares of fried bread.

No. 162. Lobster Bisque may be made same as crab, using canned lobster meat, if more convenient.

No. 163. Oyster Crabs.—These may be had of leading grocers. Heat them in melted butter for a moment only, stir carefully to keep them from sticking. Butter split crackers, toast and butter them and serve the crabs on them.

No. 164. Crab Soup, Stuffed Crab and other dishes may be prepared same as lobster.

No. 165. Lobsters.—Lobsters are in our markets the year round, but are in best condition during the late summer and early autumn months. Canned lobsters may be used in many made dishes. The ordinary cook book contains all needed information about boiling and opening them; hence, for want of space, we omit any directions of that kind, for it is the purpose of this book to supply information not to be found in the ordinary cook book.

No. 166. Boiled Lobster.—Hot. (To open and serve.) Plain lobster is usually served cold, but it is delicious served hot, although it does not present a very attractive appearance when served in this way, for to have it good and hot it must be served in the shells. Break off the claws and crack them; separate the tail part from the body, and if too large to serve in one piece, cut the tail parts in pieces crosswise, and split the body, removing the lady; then the body may be quartered, but without removing from the shell. In this way each piece can be served in the shell in a way that will admit of opening with a knife and fork. Serve with plain drawn butter only. Seasoning to taste.

No. 167. Lobster to Broil.—Of late this has been a very popular dish in the lunch rooms of Boston. First split the lobster lengthwise, which kills it at once, discard the lady and the dark vein, brush a little melted butter over the open sides and broil over a clear fire, first the shell side, then the other. Serve with melted butter.

No. 168. Lobster to Bake Whole.—Split, as for broiling, place the parts in pan open side up, sprinkle lightly with bread crumbs moistened with butter and bake twenty to thirty minutes in quick oven. The claws may be cracked and baked at the same time. Serve with melted butter, or a sauce, if preferred.

No. 169. Lobster Soup.—Chop one pound of boiled lobster meat— canned may be used—very fine. Put into double boiler, one quart each, milk and water, when it comes to a boil, stir in two tablespoons flour and add the chopped lobster, with pepper, salt and the faintest suspicion of mace, let it boil up once, add a small piece of butter, pour into tureen and serve hot.

No. 170. Lobster Chowder.—Chop one pound boiled lobster meat—canned will do—rather course. Boil one quart of milk and stir in four pounded or rolled crackers, then add the lobster. Season with salt and pepper, boil up once and serve. One small onion may be boiled, chopped and added with the lobster, if liked, but it is rich enough without.

No. 171. Astor House Lobster.—Take two live lobsters of a pound and a half each, split them, take out the meat and cut into inch pieces. Put into saucepan, one oz. of butter and thicken smooth with flour, when it melts add the lobster, stir for four or five minutes, add one gill of water, a tablespoon of catsup, a speck of cayenne, and a wine glass of sherry, simmer five minutes, add one dozen button mushrooms, cover, simmer three minutes, season and serve.

No. 172. Lobster Fricassee.—Add to the chopped meat of a boiled lobster, salt, white pepper, speck of cayenne, a tablespoon of cream and one of vinegar. Mix well; melt in a saucepan a tablespoon of butter, add the lobster and let it simmer until very hot and serve immediately.

No. 173. Lobster a la Francaise.—Remove the meat from a freshly boiled lobster and cut into small pieces about one inch square; pound the yolks of three hard-boiled eggs, mix with them half a teaspoon of salt, one teaspoon of mustard and a little cayenne, mix thoroughly, and add slowly four tablespoons of melted butter and four tablespoons vinegar; pile the lobster high in the center of a dish, pour the sauce over it, and sprinkle over the whole, parsley and lobster coral; garnish the edge of the dish with crisp yellow leaves of lettuce and slices of lemon.

No. 174. Lobster Cutlets.—Pick the meat from a large lobster and two small ones and pound it in a mortar with a part of the coral and a seasoning of pepper and salt, a blade of pounded mace, a little nutmeg and cayenne pepper; add the yolks of two well beaten eggs, the white of one and a spoonful of anchovy sauce; mix the above thoroughly and roll it out as you would pastry, with a little flour, nearly two inches thick; cut it into cutlets, brush them over with the yolk of egg, dip them into bread crumbs and fry a nice brown in butter, a spoonful of anchovy sauce and the remainder of coral; pour it into the centre of a hot dish, arrange the cutlets around it as you would cutlets of meat. Garnish each cutlet with an lobster leg.

No. 175. Stuffed Lobster.—Cut one pint boiled lobster meat into small dice shape pieces, season and mix with one cup cream and a few cracker crumbs, adding also the lobster butter. Clean the tail shells of the lobsters and fill with the mixture, cover with cracker crumbs, moisten with melted butter and bake until the crumbs are brown. Beaten egg may be mixed with the lobster, if it is desirable to make it richer, and using half wine and half cream makes it a yet more delicious dish.

No. 176. Devilled Lobster.—Cut rather fine one pound of boiled lobster meat and mix with one raw egg. Put into a saucepan one-quarter pound of butter and a tablespoon of flour, stir together until well blended, then add one gill of rich cream; season with saltspoon of salt and half as much cayenne, add a teaspoon of curry powder, one-third of a nutmeg, grated, one onion boiled to a paste, and then the lobster meat; cook two or three minutes and spread out on a platter to cool. When cool enough fill the shells with this mixture, brush over the surface with beaten egg and cover with bread crumbs, lay in a baking pan, put bits of butter on top of each, and bake a nice yellow in a brisk oven; serve hot as possible.

No. 177. Stewed Lobster.—Stir flour enough into half a pint of milk to give it a creamy thickness, heat to boiling, and remove from fire, then stir in one tablespoon of butter; drain the liquor from a one pound can of lobster, chop the meat rather coarse, and add it to the sauce, season with salt and pepper and, add a teaspoon of lemon juice, simmer ten minutes and serve hot.

No. 178. Lobster Patties.—Chop fine one pound boiled lobster meat, mash the coral smooth and mix with the lobster butter and meat, add the yolks of three hard boiled eggs grated fine, season with salt, cayenne and mace or nutmeg and a very little grated lemon peel; moisten the whole with cream, melted butter or salad oil. Put into saucepan, add a little water and let it just come to a boil, have the patty pans all ready, fill with the mixture and serve.

No. 179. Lobster Croquettes, No. 1.—Chop fine one pint boiled lobster meat, add half a pint bechamel sauce (No. 31) to which has been added the yolks of two eggs mixed in a little water, then add two tablespoons tomato sauce (No. 51,) little pepper, salt and nutmeg, set on ice to get cold. When thoroughly cold form into croquettes, roll in crumbs and beaten egg then in crumbs again and fry in hot fat. Drain and serve.

No. 180. Lobster Croquettes, No. 2.—Chop fine one pint boiled lobster meat, season with salt, mustard and cayenne, moisten with cream sauce (No. 18.) When the mixture is cool enough shape into croquettes, roll in crumbs, dip in beaten egg, roll again in crumbs and fry in hot fat, drain on paper, serve on a napkin, garnish with parsley.

No. 181. Oysters, to Fry in Crumbs.—Medium sized oysters are the best for this purpose. Season with salt and pepper and let them stand a few minutes, then roll in cracker or bread crumbs, dip in egg beaten up in milk and roll again in crumbs, fry quickly in hot fat; drain on paper as fast as taken up. Serve hot, garnished with slices of lemon. Have them as free from grease as possible.

No. 182. Oysters, to Broil.—Large oysters are preferable. Dry them in a napkin and dip each one in melted butter and dust slightly with salt and white pepper or cayenne, then roll in fine cracker dust and broil on a fine wire broiler, or they may be broiled without the crumbs, then served on well buttered soft toast spread with finely chopped celery, or mushrooms, or both, they are delicious in this way.

No. 183. Oyster Saute.—Prepare, as for frying in lard, or for broiling, and fry the oysters in butter, turning them, so as to cook both sides.

No. 184. Steamed Oysters are esteemed a delicacy served with plain, melted butter and seasoning to taste.

No. 185. Oysters Creamed on Toast.—Chop one pint oysters moderately fine, season with salt, pepper and a suspicion of mace, and put them into saucepan with melted butter. Beat the yolks of two eggs with one gill rich cream, stir in with the oysters until they begin to harden, then pour over buttered toast and serve.

No. 186. Oysters, to Parboil or Blanch.—Put them on to boil without any liquor, as enough comes from the oyster, stir or shake in a saucepan slightly at first, when the edges begin to wrinkle and the oyster looks plump they are ready for sauces and other ways of cooking, in some of which it will be noted they have to be bearded, that is, the black edges trimmed off.

No. 187. Oyster Soup.—Strain the liquor from one quart of oysters and add as much water as you have oyster liquor, and put it on to boil, skim and add the oysters and let them simmer without boiling until they begin to grow plump and the edges to wrinkle, strain out the oysters and add to the liquor one pint of boiling milk thickened with a tablespoon of butter and two of flour seasoned to taste, boil five minutes, add the oysters, which have been kept hot, and serve.

No. 188. Stewed Oysters.—Although this is a very common dish and a simple one to prepare, many people fail in their attempt to make it. Boil one quart of milk in double boiler, add one pint solid oysters, butter, salt and white pepper to taste; when the oysters begin to wrinkle serve. Some prefer to add the butter just before taking up. The stew may be poured over common crackers split, buttered and peppered, or served plain with oyster crackers, separately.

No. 189. Oysters a la Newport.—Put one tablespoon of butter in saucepan, add one pint solid oysters, a tablespoon of chopped celery, salt and white pepper to taste, cover and simmer three minutes, add a wineglass of sherry and a wineglass of cream, simmer a couple of minutes longer and serve on toast. Mushrooms instead of the celery also make a delicious dish.

No. 190. Oyster Fritters, or Oysters Fried in Batter.—For this dish the oysters may be used whole or chopped. The batter everybody has their own way of making. Drain the fritters on paper as fast as taken up, and serve, on a napkin, garnished with parsley.

No. 191. Oysters au Gratin.—Parboil one pint small oysters, or if large cut in halves or quarters, then drain; add yolks of two eggs well mixed in a little milk, to half a pint boiling cream, season with salt, pepper, and a little mace; when beginning to boil add the oysters, and mix all well together. Have some large, smooth oyster shells all cleaned, and fill them with the mixture, cover lightly with bread crumbs and melted butter on top, bake until brown.

No. 192. Scalloped Oysters.—This is a most popular dish, but the number of cooks that don't know how to make it properly is wonderful to contemplate. The following directions, strictly adhered to, cannot fail to produce satisfactory results: For one quart of solid oysters use one pint of pounded cracker crumbs, three oz. of butter, one gill of cream, half a gill of oyster liquor, pepper and salt to taste, and a suspicion of mace. Butter the baking dish and cover the bottom thickly with the pounded cracker, wet with oyster liquor and a little cream, then add a single layer of oysters, salt and pepper and a bit of butter on each oyster, then more crumbs, oysters and so on, until the dish is full, the top layer being crumbs, dotted over with bits of butter. Set in the oven with a plate or other cover and bake until the juice bubbles up to the top, then remove the cover and pour over the whole one glass of sherry or Maderia wine and return to the oven to brown slightly. The wine may be omitted if objectionable, but we know of no dish where a glass of wine so enhances its flavor.

No. 193. Oyster Pie.—Line a deep dish with a good puff paste, not too rich, roll out upper crust and lay on plate, just the size of pie dish, set it on top of the dish and put it into the oven, as the crust must be nearly cooked before the oysters are put in, for they require less cooking than the crust. While the crust is baking strain the liquor from the oysters and thicken with yolks of eggs boiled hard and grated (three eggs for one quart of oysters) add two tablespoons butter and the same of cracker crumbs, season with salt, pepper and nutmeg or mace. Let the liquor just boil, slip in the oysters, let it boil up once, then stir, remove plate with the crust, pour the oysters and hot liquor into the pie dish, put the top crust on and return to oven for five minutes.

No. 194. Oyster Patties.—Cut one quart of oysters into small pieces and stir into one cup rich drawn butter based on milk, season to taste, cook five minutes, fill the patty cases, heat two minutes and serve.

No. 195. Oyster Croquettes.—Parboil one pint of oysters, drain and chop, moisten with a thick cream sauce and the oyster liquor, add one teaspoon chopped parsley and bread or cracker crumbs sufficient to make the mixture firm enough to shape, season with salt, pepper and a little onion juice. Let the mixture get cold, then shape into croquettes and fry in hot fat in a frying basket if you have it, drain and serve on a hot napkin.

No. 196. Mayonnaise Dressing.—Set a bowl into cracked ice, and into it put yolks of three raw eggs, one tablespoon of dry mustard, one of sugar, speck of cayenne, and saltspoon of salt; beat all together with a good egg beater until light and thick, then add one pint of oil, beginning with a few drops at a time. When the dressing is quite hard add two table spoons of vinegar and the juice of one lemon, beating all the while; if too thick add more vinegar. When of right consistency set away to keep cool, and do not pour over the lobster until just before serving.

No. 197. Mayonnaise Dressing.—(Red.) The red mayonnaise is made by adding a liberal quantity of lobster coral, juice of boiled beets or tomato juice to the common mayonnaise.

No. 198. Mayonnaise Dressing.—(Green.) The green mayonnaise is made by coloring with the water in which spinach has been boiled. The colored mayonnaise is chiefly used in fish and vegetable salads.

No. 199. Cream Dressing for Salads.—Beat together thoroughly three raw eggs and six tablespoons of cream, three tablespoons melted butter, one teaspoon salt, one of dry mustard, half a teaspoon black pepper, and one teacup vinegar. Heat, stirring constantly, until it thickens like boiled custard, but it must not boil. When cold mix with salad.

No. 200. Piquante Salad Dressing.—Mix yolks of two hard boiled eggs and two raw eggs, add one teaspoon each cream and oil, half a teaspoon horseradish, and vinegar enough to reduce to consistency of cream. This is very good for fish salads, for fish balls, and broiled, smoked or salted fish of all kinds.

No. 201. French Salad Dressing.—To one teaspoon of salt and half as much pepper, add one tablespoon of oil, and mix thoroughly, adding a few drops extract of onion, then add more oil and vinegar until the mixture is of desired consistency.

No. 202. Sardine Salad Dressing.—Bruise to a paste four boneless sardines, add the yolks of four hard boiled eggs, and bruise all together thoroughly; add this mixture to any mayonnaise dressing and serve on fish salads.

No. 203. Lobster Salad.—Extract the meat from a couple of boiled lobsters weighing two pounds each, cut it into rather coarse pieces and set it on the ice to cool. Separate the tender leaves of two heads of lettuce, and put them in layers on the salad dish and put this on the ice also. When ready to serve mix a part of the mayonnaise dressing (No. 208) with the lobster meat and put it on the lettuce, pouring the remainder of the dressing over the whole and sprinkling the top with grated lobster coral if you have it. Any other mayonnaise or salad dressing may be used.

No. 204. Crab Salad.—Prepare the meat and use same dressing as for lobster.

No. 205. Fish Salad.—Reduce one quart cold cooked fish to flakes, rejecting bones, skin and liquor, arrange on a bed of lettuce with a sardine or piquante dressing; garnish with sliced cucumber or boiled beets, or both.

No. 206. Salmon Salad.—May be made same as lobster salad, using either cold boiled fresh salmon, or canned salmon. In either case remove all bones, skin or other matter than the clear meat, which must be drained entirely free from any liquid matter.

No. 207. Shrimp Salad.—Chop together, one cup celery and one cup lettuce; arrange a bed of lettuce leaves on shallow dish; season the chopped celery and lettuce with salt, pepper and vinegar, add a little melted butter, mix one can of shrimps and place on the lettuce leaves. Just before serving, pour over it a French dressing (No. 201) and sprinkle on a few capers.

No. 208. Oyster Salad.—Cook one quart of oysters in their own liquor, drain and chop rather coarsely together with six quahogs chopped fine, add one cup chopped celery and one small onion chopped fine, mix thoroughly with mustard, oil, salt, pepper and vinegar, arrange on a bed of lettuce and pour over the salad a cream dressing (No. 199.)

No. 209. Eels to Fry.—Cut skinned eels into desired lengths, roll in crumbs dipped in egg or without, and fry in hot fat.

No. 210. Eels to Broil.—We know of no better way to cook this often despised but really delicious fish, and although it need not necessarily be skinned for that purpose, we much prefer it in that way, then when split it can be nicely browned on both sides. Butter, pepper and salt are the only condiments needed to bring out its delicate flavor. Large eels are always the best, and particularly so for broiling.

No. 211. Eels Fricasseed.—Cut three pounds of skinned eels into three inch lengths, put them into a saucepan and cover with Rhine wine or two-thirds water and one-third vinegar, add fifteen oysters, two slices of lemon, a bouquet of herbs, one onion, quartered, six cloves, three stalks of celery, pinch of cayenne, and salt to taste. Stew the eels forty-five minutes, very slowly, then remove them from the saucepan and strain the liquor, then heat in this for a few minutes a gill of cream and an ounce of butter rolled in flour, simmering gently, pour over fish and serve. If you are prejudiced against eels your prejudice will vanish once you have partaken of this delicious dish. Small skinned fish may be cooked in almost any way directed for eels.

No. 212. Eels Stewed.—Cut two pounds skinned eels into three inch pieces; rub inside and out with salt and let them stand one hour, then parboil. Boil one onion in a quart of milk, take out the onion, drain the eels and add to the milk. Season with half a teaspoon of chopped parsley, salt, pepper and a very little mace. Simmer until the flesh separates from the bones. Thicken the gravy with butter and flour, pour over eels and serve.

No. 213. Eels to Stew.—Take two pounds skinned eels, cut in short pieces and soak in strong salted water one hour; dry them and fry them brown. Put one pint stock (No. 14) in saucepan with one gill port wine, one teaspoon anchovy essence, juice of half a lemon, salt, cayenne and powdered mace; when hot put in the eels and stew gently for half an hour. Serve with the gravy poured over them.

No. 214. Eels Collared.—Take an eel weighing two pounds, skin, split and take out back bone; on the inside sprinkle with salt, pepper, pounded mace, ground cloves, ground allspice, a tablespoon of powdered sage and teaspoon of powdered sweet marjoram, all well mixed. Roll up the eel, beginning at the widest end, and bind with a piece of tape; boil in salted water and a little vinegar until tender. Serve whole, or in slices, with or without sauce.

No. 215. Eels en Matelote.—Take two pounds skinned eels and cut into three lengths, sprinkle salt inside and out and let them stand one hour, then wipe dry without washing, put them to cook in a stewpan with one-third red wine and two-thirds water, two bay leaves, a little thyme, three cloves, a blade of mace, pepper and salt, simmer gently thirty to forty minutes, not long enough to let them break to pieces, remove to serving dish and keep hot; strain the liquid, add one tablespoon of brandy, and three of cream, heat hot and pour over the eels, which should be served hot.

No. 216. Black Bass, Burgundy Sauce.—Put four pounds of fish in kettle with half a bottle of claret and let it simmer half an hour. Take half a pint of Spanish sauce (No. 37) and put in a saucepan with two wine glasses red wine, reduce one quarter and serve with the fish. Almost any kind of fresh water fish may be cooked and served in this way.

No. 217. Boiled Striped Bass.—Newport style. Put six pounds of fish in cold water, enough to cover, with one gill of claret wine, teaspoon salt, one onion, one large pepper and blade of mace. Heat slowly at first, boil half an hour, make a drawn butter, using the fish liquor and adding juice of one lemon. Dish the bass on a napkin, garnish with sliced lemon. Serve the sauce in tureen. Halibut, sword-fish and other large, firm-meated fish are adapted to this way of cooking.

No. 218. Baked Bluefish, Tomato Sauce.—Prepare a fish of about four pounds and put it in buttered pan, cover with tomato pulp, sprinkle liberally with bread crumbs and dot with bits of butter. Place in oven for about forty minutes, until the flesh begins to separate from the back bone, or can be easily detached from it. Serve with tomato sauce (No. 52) poured around the fish. Bonita, Spanish mackerel and fish of a similar kind are all good served with a tomato sauce.

No. 219. Carp to Cook.—This fish has recently been naturalized in American waters and should in time become abundant and cheap, from the fact that it multiplys rapidly, acquires a large size and flourishes in waters where other fish would speedily become extinct. The scales are said to be eatable, and in cleaning the fish these should not be removed, but the fish should be scoured in salted water. There seems to be a diversity of opinion concerning its flavor, but in the report of the U. S. Fish Commission we find it highly praised. The better way to cook this fish is to boil or bake, and the same recipes given for bass, sheepshead, or similar fish, are well suited to the carp.

No. 220. Fresh Cod Cheeks and Tongues.—These are very nice fried, either plain or rolled in crumbs or beaten egg.

No. 221. Fillets of Cod a la Regence.—Butter a tin dish, lay on it three slices of cod an inch thick, pour over them one glass white wine, cover with a buttered paper and bake in moderate oven fifteen minutes. Reduce another glass of wine in a saucepan by simmering, add to it half a pint of white sauce (No. 19) twelve oysters, bearded and blanched, twelve small quenelles (No. 90) and twelve button mushrooms. Season with pepper and salt. Simmer one minute only. Place the slices of fish on a hot dish, pour the sauce over them, group the oysters, mushrooms and quenelles in the corners of the dish.

No. 222. Cod Steaks a la Cardinal.—Cut about three pounds of fine fresh codfish into slices quite an inch thick; sprinkle these well with salt, pepper and lemon juice, and fasten each slice with a small skewer, so as to make it into a neat shape. Brush the fish over entirely with warmed butter, then lay it at the bottom of a large saucepan, pour over it about a breakfast cupful of very good white stock, and cover closely, first with buttered paper, then with the pan lid. Simmer gently from 20 to 25 minutes, then take skewers and arrange the fish neatly on a hot dish; pour over it some well made tomato sauce, flavored with essence of anchovy, garnish round the edge of dish with sprigs of fresh parsley and slices of lemon cut in pretty, fanciful shapes, and serve just as hot as possible.

No. 223. Fillet of Flounder a la Normandy.—Prepare the fillets and lay in a buttered baking pan, season with salt and pepper, dredge with flour, moisten with brown stock, adding a teaspoon of lemon juice, bake twenty minutes, baste once or twice, lay the fillets on serving dish, pour over them Normandy sauce (No. 49) garnish with slices of lemon.

No. 224. Baked Haddock.—Stuff with a dressing (No. 86) baste the fish well with butter, put a cup of water into the pan and bake in a moderate oven one hour, basting often; just before taking up sprinkle a tablespoon of fine cracker crumbs over the fish and let it remain in the oven long enough to brown them delicately. Put the fish on a warm platter, add water and thickening to the gravy and serve in gravy tureen. Garnish with parsley and sliced lemon. A plain and simple method for baking cod or any white-meated fish.

No. 225. Cod Boiled, Oyster Sauce.—Boil a fish or the head and shoulders, stuffed or not, in salted water, 30 minutes for six pounds. Serve on a napkin garnished with parsley or slices of hard boiled eggs, and serve with an oyster sauce. A plain, simple way to boil any kind of fish. Serve any sauce to suit.

No. 226. Baked Halibut.—Take a square piece of fish, weighing about five pounds, lay it in salted water for about five hours, then wipe dry and place it in the dripping pan with a few very thin slices of salt pork on top. Bake one hour, or until the fish is easily separated from the bone, or cracks open; baste with melted butter and water. Stir into the gravy one tablespoon Worcestershire sauce, juice of one lemon, seasoning to suit, and thicken. Dish the fish on a napkin and serve the gravy separately, garnish with slices of hard-boiled eggs.

No. 227. Chicken Halibut aux Fine Herbs.—Chop a little parsley, six mushrooms and a shallot, adding to them a little salt, pepper and nutmeg; place all in a saucepan and simmer five minutes with half a pint of port wine. Pour all these ingredients into a shallow dish and place on top four pounds of chicken halibut. Bake in moderate oven for about thirty minutes, basting with the liquor occasionally. Put half a pint of Spanish sauce (No. 37) in another saucepan and reduce for seven or eight minutes, adding juice of a lemon, serve poured around the fish.

No. 228. Smelts Baked.—Dip in beaten egg, roll in cracker crumbs, season with salt, pepper and a little nutmeg, lay on a sheet of buttered paper in a buttered baking pan, put a piece of butter on each fish and bake a delicate brown; serve on a hot dish, garnished with slices of lemon and parsley.

No. 229. Halibut a la Royale.—Six pounds fish in one piece, half a cup of bread crumbs, two slices fat, salt pork, two teaspoons essence anchovy, one quarter cup melted butter, one cup boiling water, juice of one lemon, pepper and salt. Lay the fish in salted water for two hours, wipe and make incisions each side of back bone and put in a dressing (No. 84.) Pour into bottom of neat baking dish the butter, hot water, lemon juice and anchovy essence. Lay in the fish, cover and bake one hour, basting often, send to table in the dish.

No. 230. Halibut, Sauce Supreme.—Cut four pounds of halibut in square pieces one inch thick, soak one hour in Maderia or sherry wine, turning them over once in fifteen minutes. Then put them into a saucepan with two oz. melted butter, add salt and pepper; simmer five minutes, then send to the oven for twenty minutes. Arrange the fish on a dish and pour over it a sauce supreme. Cook sword fish, flounders or bass in the same way. Striped bass, deep sea flounders, sword fish and other coarse grained fish may be cooked in any way directed for the halibut.

No. 231. Baked Herring.—Split two herring, remove heads, tails and backbone, lay one fish skin side down, mix together one desertspoon finely chopped parsley, one small onion, chopped, and half a teaspoon each thyme and marjoram, powdered, a few bread crumbs, with salt and pepper, and sprinkle over the fish, lay the other fish on top, skin side up, and pour over them melted butter, cover and bake half an hour, watching and basting. Mackerel, alewives and porgies may be cooked in the same way.

No. 232. Grilled Herring.—To grill is to broil on the gridiron. Do not split the fish, but score them slightly at the sides, grease the gridiron with butter, turn the fish often while grilling, brown them evenly all over, dish on a hot platter and pour over them a sauce made of two ounces butter, one teaspoon flour, two of vinegar, four of French mustard, half a gill of water, pepper and salt. Heat all together, smooth, thicken and boil five minutes, garnish with parsley. Alewives, menhaden and small shad can be cooked in the same way.

No. 233. King Fish, Sherry Sauce.—Split in two four medium size fish, take out the backbone and broil over a gentle fire, when done put half a pint of Spanish sauce (No. 37) in saucepan, add wineglass of sherry wine, boil fifteen minutes, pour around the fish and serve. A good way to cook butter-fish, tautog, or blackfish.

No. 234. Mackerel to Broil.—This is undoubtedly the best way to cook a fresh mackerel, especially if it is fat, and it should be in the fall. Serve basted with cream or melted butter, seasoned to taste, or with a maitre d'hotel butter (No. 32,) or a sauce tartare (No. 44.) Mackerel may also be cooked in any way a shad is cooked. Very small mackerel may be cooked the same as smelts.

No. 235. Perch to Cook.—Perch of all kinds are best fried, but may be cooked in any way recommended for small fish of other kinds. Some varieties are rather tasteless, and these should be served according to some of the rich stews, fricassees, &c., mentioned under the head of fish cookery in general.

No. 236. Pickerel Baked.—Score back and thick parts of sides, baste well with flour, butter, pepper and salt, sprinkle lightly with lemon juice and lay in dripping pan with two tablespoons of water, baste occasionally, adding more water if needed; bake from thirty to fifty minutes, according to size. Make a drawn butter sauce based on the fish gravy, add a pinch of cayenne, pour over fish and serve.

No. 237. Ray with Caper Sauce.—Put the fish in kettle with one sliced carrot, one sliced onion, three cloves of garlic, six bay leaves, six cloves, six branches thyme, four parsley roots, and cover the fish with half a bottle white wine and one quart consomme (No. 14,) when it comes to a boil remove the fish to baking pan and cook slowly for one hour, basting freely with the liquor in which it was boiled. Serve with a sauce made from the gravy, adding capers, thickening and seasoning to taste. Striped bass, deep sea flounders and other coarse-meated fish may be cooked by the recipes given for cooking the ray.

No. 238. Salmon Cutlets, Herb Sauce.—Cut the salmon in slices an inch thick and about three inches square, or of a diamond shape. Chop fine half a dozen button onions, a little parsley and thyme, add pepper, salt and a dash of mace or nutmeg. Put these ingredients in saucepan with a little water and a glass of wine; heat for about five minutes. Put all in a suitable dish for baking, on top put the cutlets, cover and bake half an hour, basting freely from time to time with the liquid. When done, arrange the fish on a hot platter, add another glass of wine to the gravy, with the juice of a lemon and pour all over the fish and serve. Half a dozen mushrooms chopped and put in with the herbs will be found an improvement.

No. 239. Trout Baked, Herb Sauce.—Clean, wash and dry six trout of about one quarter pound each. Place them on a buttered dish, adding half a glass of white wine and one finely chopped shallot. Cook ten minutes, then put the gravy in a saucepan with tablespoon of cooked herbs, moistening with half a pint of sauce allemande (No. 34.) Reduce gravy one half and pour it over the trout with the juice of half a lemon and serve.

No. 240. Baked Salmon Trout with Cream Gravy.—Wipe dry and lay in pan with just enough water to keep from scorching. If large, score the back, but not the sides, bake slowly from three quarters to one hour, basting with butter and water. Into a cup of rich cream stir three or four tablespoons boiling water (or cream will clot when heated,) into this stir gently two tablespoons melted butter and a little chopped parsley. Put this into milk boiler or farina kettle, or any vessel you can set into another, half filled with boiling water to prevent sauce from burning; add the cream and butter to the gravy from the dripping pan in which fish was baked; lay the trout on a hot platter and let the gravy boil up once, then pour over the fish; garnish with sprigs of parsley. Use no spiced sauces and very little salt. This creamed gravy may be used for various kinds of boiled and baked fish.

No. 241. Baked Shad.—Stuff with dressing (No. 84,) rub the fish well with flour, lay in pan with a very few thin slices of pork on top. Bake a medium size fish forty minutes, add a little hot water, butter, pepper and salt to the gravy; boil up and serve in gravy tureen. Garnish the fish with sprigs of parsley. A tablespoon of anchovy sauce, or a glass of wine, is a decided improvement in making the gravy.

No. 242. Fillets of Shad with Mushrooms.—Prepare the fillets in the usual way, cutting in equal size and shape; put them on a plate, skin side down, and sprinkle each with a little salt, pepper, lemon juice and chopped parsley; let them remain in this condition fifteen minutes, then put them into a saucepan with a glass of white wine and an oz. of butter. Have ready a few stewed mushrooms, and when the fish are done remove them to a hot platter; put the mushrooms into the fish gravy, add another glass of wine and a wineglass of cream, simmer a minute and pour over the fish. If this doesn't go to the right spot there is something the matter with the fish, the mushrooms, or the one who partakes of it.

No. 243. Baked Tautog, or Black Fish.—The tautog is a very nice fish. It is in best condition in the fall, but it is good at all times. In New York markets it is best known as the black fish. About Buzzard's Bay and Vineyard Sound, where it is very plenty, it is generally called tautog. It is a difficult fish to scale, but the operation is made easier by pouring boiling water over it, but it must not soak in the hot water for an instant. It may be skinned for baking, in which case it is better to cover it with a buttered paper while baking, removing the paper in time to brown the fish before taking from the oven. The fish should be scored before baking and narrow strips of fat pork inserted in the gashes made. In May and June always save the roe to this fish—it may be baked with the fish, or fried separately—it is too good to be wasted. Make a dressing as for any fish, and prepare the gravy in the usual way.

No. 244. Salmon.—The ordinary cook book is full pf recipes for cooking this king of fishes, hence we have given it less attention than those varieties neglected by these books. There is no better way to cook this delicious fish than to boil, and it should be served with a simple sauce. Some of the recipes for turbot, trout or sole may be used for cooking salmon. That for salmon trout (No. 240) will be found just the thing for the land locked salmon.

No. 245. Sheepshead a la Creole.—The sheepshead is one of the best of our saltwater fishes; it is not so plenty as formerly, but some seasons it is quite plenty in our markets. To cook, put one chopped onion and one chopped green pepper (seed extracted) in a stewpan, and brown in half a gill of oil for five minutes; add one tomato sliced, four sliced mushrooms, a good bouquet of herbs and a clove of garlic; season with salt and pepper and moisten with half a pint of sauce allemande. Cut three pounds of fish into slices, lay them flat in the stewpan with three tablespoons of mushroom liquor, and cook for one hour on a slow fire. When ready to serve, sprinkle over with a tablespoon of chopped parsley and decorate with six heart-shaped croutons.

No. 246. Trout a la Chambord.—Make a forcemeat with one pound of firm, fresh fish, remove the skin and bones, pound well in a mortar, adding the whites of three eggs, a little at a time; when well pounded add half a pint of cream, half a teaspoon of salt and a little white pepper and nutmeg; mix well and use a portion of it for stuffing three trout of half a pound each; butter well a deep baking dish and lay in the trout, add half a glass of white wine, a bouquet of herbs, salt and pepper; bake fifteen minutes, basting often; take up the fish and put them on a dish to keep hot, remove the gravy to a saucepan, add one truffle and four mushrooms, sliced, (take out the bouquet) also a glass of wine; heat hot and pour over the fish, decorate with six quenelles made from the remaining forcemeat.

No. 247. Sturgeon Roasted.—Take a piece of fish that is adapted to stuffing, make a dressing (No. 89.) Rub well inside and out with salt, butter and pepper; stuff and sew up, or bind firmly, and lay in baking pan with a very little water, cover with paper until nearly done, then remove paper and sprinkle a few bread crumbs over the fish and let it brown nicely. Serve with plain butter and flour added to the fish gravy. If you have a piece to roast that will not admit of stuffing, prepare some forcemeat balls (No. 89) and bake beside the fish. Some cook books recommend removing the back bone and inserting the dressing in the space thus obtained, but as the sturgeon has no bones whatever, this might prove a difficult thing to do.

No. 248. Brochet of Smelts.—Spread melted butter in bottom of shallow baking dish, dredge with raspings of bread, season with salt, pepper, chopped parsley and shallots; put in a laying of fish and pour over it a glass of wine and a teaspoon of anchovy sauce; cover with melted butter and bread raspings, and bake in oven fifteen minutes. Serve hot; arrange the fish on a napkin, heads to heads, in center of dish, or lay them all one way in rows, each row overlapping the next about two thirds the length of fish. Garnish with quartered lemon and fried parsley.

No. 249. Trout a la Genevoise.—Cut the heads off four little trout and put the fish in an earthen pot for four hours, with a little thyme, four bay leaves, two shallots cut in pieces, five branches of parsley, little pepper and salt and the juice of two lemons; then take out the fish and put them in a saucepan with a chopped onion, a clove of garlic and enough red wine to cover the fish; boil gently for twenty minutes; then strain the liquid in stone pot and add one half of it to half a pint of Spanish sauce (No. 37) and boil for one hour; then add four chopped mushrooms and truffles and a little parsley. Dish the trout, garnish with parsley and serve the sauce separately.

No. 250. Stewed Trout.—Take two trout of a pound each and lay them in a saucepan with half an onion sliced thin, a little chopped parsley, two cloves, one blade of mace, two bay leaves, a little thyme, salt and pepper, one pint white stock (No. 14) and wineglass port wine; simmer gently half an hour, or more, if not quite done. Dish the trout, strain the gravy, thicken with butter and flour, stirring over sharp fire five minutes, pour over fish and serve.

No. 251. Brook Trout.—Put a trout of four pounds in fish kettle with four oz. of salt; when beginning to boil, set the kettle on the back of the range for twenty-five minutes. Parboil the roes of a shad in salted water, drain and cut them in small pieces, and also a dozen mushrooms, add these with the juice of a lemon to one pint of sauce allemande (No. 34) and boil ten minutes. Serve the fish garnished with sprigs of parsley and the sauce in a tureen.

No. 252. Scallops of Trout.—Take a medium size trout and cut into slices one inch thick, put into a saucepan with a little melted butter, add salt, white pepper and the juice of a lemon; when done on one side, turn and cook the other. Mash some boiled potatoes and with them form a border on a platter that can go to the oven; moisten the potatoes lightly with melted butter and brown in the oven; when done arrange the scallops in the center of the potato border and pour over it a sauce bechamel (No. 31.)

No. 253. Boiled Turbot.—Soak the fish first in salted water to take off slime, do not cut off fins; when clean make an incision down the middle of the back to prevent skin on the other side from cracking, rub it over with lemon and lay it in kettle of cold water; after it gets to boiling let it boil slowly; when done, drain well and lay on hot napkin; rub a little lobster coral through a sieve, sprinkle it over fish and garnish with sprigs of parsley and sliced lemon. Serve with lobster (No. 30) or shrimp sauce, or with plain drawn butter. The old fashioned way of dishing this fish is white side up, but now usually the dark side up.

1. Fish Balls.—3 pints of potatoes (measured after being pared and cut into pieces), 1 package of Favorite brand Picked codfish, 1 small onion (cut into pieces), 1 tablespoonful of butter, 1 large or two small eggs. Boil the potatoes and onion until soft, drain off all the water and mash until free from lumps. Turn the fish into a napkin and pour through it about one pint of cold water and squeeze. Mix with the potato, using a fork as it makes it lighter, add the butter and the beaten egg; now taste and if not salt enough add a little. Take up by the spoonful and drop into deep fat which is hot enough to brown a piece of bread in 40 seconds, fry until a golden brown (about 1 minute,) drain on soft paper. This makes twenty medium size fish balls. The onion can be omitted if the flavor is not liked.

2. Fish Balls.—Take one pint bowl of Diamond Wedge brand codfish picked very fine, 2 pint bowls whole raw potatoes sliced thickly, put them together in plenty of cold water and boil until potatoes are thoroughly cooked; remove from the fire and drain off all the water, mash them with a potato masher, add piece of butter size of an egg, one well beaten egg, and three teaspoonfuls of cream or rich milk. Flour your hands and make into balls or cakes. Put an ounce of butter and lard into a frying pan, when hot put in the balls and fry a nice brown. Do not freshen the fish before boiling with the potatoes. Many cooks fry them in a quantity of lard similar to boiled doughnuts.

3. "Diamond Wedge" Fish Balls.—One pint of raw potatoes, cut in pieces; one cup of "Diamond Wedge" Codfish. Boil together until potatoes are tender, then draw off the water and mash, beating well together; add one tablespoonful of butter, one egg and a little pepper. Shape into small balls and fry in hot lard.

4. Fish Balls.—To one-half pound package "Gold Wedge Brand" Fibered Codfish add double quantity mashed potatoes. Saturate the codfish with cold water slightly, and strain through a cloth (requires no soaking.) Mix thoroughly with the potatoes; add one tablespoonful of butter and a little pepper. Shape into small balls and fry in hot lard.

The addition of an egg to the above receipt improves it very much.

For Creamed Codfish.—Saturate as above; to a gill or cup of fish add two of milk and one tablespoonful of butter. Let it come to a boil; then add one teaspoonful cornstarch and one egg well beaten. Served on toast it makes a delicious dish.

Fish Sauce.—Rub smooth 2 tablespoons of butter with 1 of flour, stir into a pint of boiling milk, let it simmer a few minutes; have ready in the sauce dish a hard boiled egg, cut fine; pour the sauce over it.

A Nice Relish for Breakfast or Tea, Broiled Smoked Halibut.—Remove the skin and soak over night with the skin side downward. Broil and garnish with butter and serve hot.

Stewed Codfish (Salt).—Take a thick white piece of Diamond Wedge salt codfish, lay it in cold water for a few minutes to soften it a little, enough to make it more easily to be picked up. Shred it in very small bits, put it over the fire in a stewpan with cold water; let it come to a boil, turn off this water carefully, and add a pint of milk to the fish, or more according to quantity. Set it over the fire again and let it boil slowly about three minutes, now add a good sized piece of butter, a shake of pepper and a thickening of a tablespoonful of flour in enough cold milk to make a cream. Stew five minutes longer, and just before serving stir in two well beaten eggs. The eggs are an addition that can be dispensed with, however, as it is very good without them. An excellent breakfast dish.

Codfish a la Mode.—Pick up a teacup full of Diamond Wedge salt codfish very fine, and freshen—the dessicated is nice to use; two cups of mashed potatoes, one pint cream or milk, two well beaten eggs, half cup of butter, salt and pepper; mix, bake in an earthen baking dish from twenty to twenty-five minutes; serve in the same dish placed on a small platter, covered with a napkin.

Fillet of Sole Baked.—Cut a fish of four pounds into fillets, about five inches long by four inches wide, each end tapering to a point. Put these in buttered pan, cover with sauce allemande (No. 34) and sprinkle with bread crumbs and dot with bits of butter. Bake until well browned. Add a wine glass of sherry to half a pint of sauce allemande, boil ten minutes and pour around the fish and serve.

For Escalloped Codfish.—Freshen one-half pound package of Shute & Merchant's Fibered Codfish by soaking three minutes in cold water, then add one pint of cracker crumbs, one tablespoonful of butter and four eggs, beaten light. Season to taste, bake until brown, serve hot.

FOOTNOTES

[1] **Note.**—Originally fish boiled in sea water, but now applied to fish boiled in salt water with acids, spices or herbs.

INDEX

A

No.
Alewives <u>231-232</u>

B

Black Bass, Burgundy Sauce <u>216</u>
Bluefish, Tomato Sauce <u>218</u>
Bonita <u>216</u>
Butter Fish <u>233</u>

C

Carp to Cook <u>219</u>
Chub   " <u>212</u>
Clam Bisque <u>130</u>
    " Chowder <u>125-126</u>
    " Croquettes <u>133</u>
    " Fritters <u>139</u>
    " Soup <u>124</u>
    " Water <u>129</u>
Clams a la Creole <u>135</u>
    "   " Creme <u>127</u>
    " au Gratin <u>134</u>
    " Fried <u>137</u>
    " Hustled <u>123</u>
    " on Toast <u>136</u>
    " Puree of <u>131</u>
    " Round or Quahogs <u>141</u>
    " Scalloped <u>132-138</u>
    " Soft Stewed <u>140</u>
    " Steamed <u>128</u>
Cod Boiled, Oyster Sauce <u>225</u>
    " Cheeks and Tongues <u>220</u>
    " Fillets a la Regence <u>221</u>

CPSIA information can be obtained
at www.ICGtesting.com
Printed in the USA
BVHW020803190423
662564BV00022B/767